New (10/01)

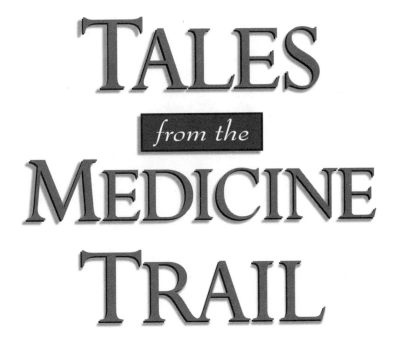

TALES
from the
MEDICINE
TRAIL

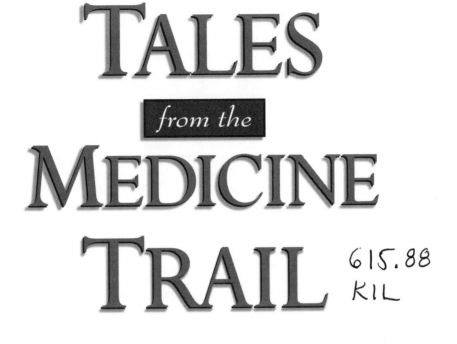

TALES *from the* MEDICINE TRAIL

Tracking down the health secrets of shamans, herbalists, mystics, yogis, and other healers

Chris Kilham, Medicine Hunter

RODALE

REACH™

An Imprint of Rodale Books

Notice

This book is meant to increase your knowledge in the use of plants for medicinal purposes. It is not intended to be used as a medical manual. The information given here is designed to help you make informed decisions about your health. It should in no way be used as a substitute for consultation with your medical doctor or other health care professional. Further, it is not intended as a substitute for any treatment that may have been prescribed by your doctor. We urge you to seek the best medical resources available to help you make informed medical decisions.

© 2000 by Christopher S. Kilham
Illustrations © by Scott MacNeill

Printed in the United States of America on acid-free ∞, recycled paper ♲

Interior Designer: Joanna Williams
Cover Designer: Christopher Rhoads
Cover Photographs: Kurt Wilson/Rodale Images, PhotoDisc (lotus flower, compass, and map)
Interior Photographs: Christopher S. Kilham
Illustrator: Scott MacNeill

Library of Congress Cataloging-in-Publication Data

Kilham, Christopher.
    Tales from the medicine trail : tracking down the health secrets of shamans, herbalists, mystics, yogis, and other healers / Chris Kilham.
        p.   cm.
    Includes index.
    ISBN 1–57954–185–2 hardcover
    1. Alternative medicine.   2. Healers.   3. Shamans.   I. Title.
R733 .K54   2000
615.88—dc21   00–025878

Distributed to the book trade by St. Martin's Press

2   4   6   8   10   9   7   5   3   hardcover

Visit us on the Web at www.rodalebooks.com, or call us toll-free at (800) 848-4735.

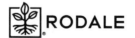

CONTENTS

On the Maca Trail

Nights of Kava

ACKNOWLEDGMENTS

Many people have made contributions to this book or have been supportive through the process of writing. First and foremost, I wish to thank my wife, Shahannah, who is a terrific traveling companion on the trail and has been helpful in the field and at home. Thanks to my mother, Elizabeth Kilham, whose unwavering support and enthusiasm matter greatly. Thanks also to Craig Weatherby, who has listened to every story dozens of times.

Thanks to Paul and Natalie Koether at PureWorld for their support of my kava and maca research, and the extensive travel and time both have entailed. Thanks to Mel Rich of Great Earth for sponsoring some of my Amazon research, and to Nutraceutical Corporation for supporting further work in the Amazon. Thanks to Muhammed Majeed of Sabinsa Corporation for valuable assistance in India. To Bill and Kahala Ann Gibson, thank you for sponsoring awa research in Hawaii. Thanks also to Ken Hakuta and the AllHerb.com Foundation for a grant supporting further kava research in Vanuatu.

Special thanks to Cynthia Hill and Nancy Morgan of Lincoln Travel, who get us there and back expertly and with great care.

Thanks to Nancy Hancock, my editor at Rodale, for working with me with talent, humor, and good cheer.

Finally, thanks to all the people on the medicine trail who appear on these pages.

PREFACE

Ipupiara the shaman sat beating a drum. The steady toomp-toomp-toomp of the taut animal-skin head resonated with a mesmerizing tone. As I relaxed with every beat, I had the odd sensation of slipping out of the borders of my body. Ipupiara began to chant softly and passionately in a high, strained voice, propitiating the gods of heaven and earth in the ancient tribal language of the Amazonian Eur Eu Wa Wa, the people born of the stars. His chanting, accompanied by the round, open beat of the drum, conjured twilight.

"On this path of life that you are traveling," Ipupiara said in a gentle, measured tone, "you must find your own way and seek the wisdom of all the spirits, who are here to assist you. This is your quest, to receive teachings that will guide you to fulfill your purpose, whatever that purpose may be."

As Ipupiara spoke, he continued to beat the drum. I had the impression that each beat was a mighty beast of burden carrying on its back ponderous words of great and lasting import. In my mind, the humpy herd of drumbeats carried Ipupiara's language across a landscape until it disappeared from view on a faraway horizon.

Ipupiara resumed chanting, a gentle plaintive call. The tone and cadence of his voice wove an inviting spell. I felt as though I were being washed away in a stream. All sensation of lying on the ground, or of being within the confines of a body, dissolved. Occasionally a distant toomp of a drumbeat would hoof slowly toward the periphery of my awareness, and then away.

In one quickening moment I became keenly lucid. I gathered myself upright, imbued with vibrant energy. Turning to my left, I admired with curiosity the mouth of a cave. The opening was surrounded by solid rock, on which moss grew and vines crept. The tunnel appeared to go deep into the earth. I knew that it was important for me to travel into the cave, and that if I remained vigilant and focused in my intent, I would receive a valuable teaching.

The floor of the cave was composed of smooth, rounded stones, which were covered with dew and satisfying to walk upon. I could stand fully upright and stretch my arms out far to the sides, touching neither roof nor walls, which were coated with moist lichen. As I glided deep into the cave, the light grew dim. But I found myself surrounded by a fine layer of luminous blue mist, helping me onward far into the interior of the underground chamber.

I felt at ease, at home with the rock and earth and air and dampness. As I ghosted deeper into the cave, I spied a glimmering light in the distance, and to this light I drew myself. Eventually I came to an opening, where light shone and water fell in a brilliant cascade. I admired the beautiful scene for a little while, but then headed back through the long, deep cave the way I'd come. I was searching for a teaching.

Just as I had retraced most of the tunnel, a small gray owl

flew close over my head and glided quickly out of the mouth of the cave. Behind me and to my left stalked a great tan cougar. The cat prowled casually by, muscular shoulders working up and down.

Ipupiara's voice called out from very far away, "Ask him for the teaching." I turned to the cat. "Do you have a teaching for me?" The powerful feline's head turned up, amber eyes locking onto mine. And then he spoke. "You must journey to other worlds, and then tell people what you saw."

INTRODUCTION

Native people refer to treading the path of healing knowledge as walking the medicine trail. I like that description because it gives a sense of purpose and conveys that the accumulation of knowledge is in fact a journey. This certainly is true in my line of work as a medicine hunter. In the course of researching traditional medicines, I have been to some remarkable places around the world, met many highly talented and unusual people, and learned about the vast and fascinating realm of natural healing, especially the use of beneficial plants of all kinds. In the course of traveling along the medicine trail, I have come to believe that plants must be restored to their proper place in health care, as primary medicines for treating illness and promoting well-being.

You may be surprised to learn that a full 85 percent of the world's population turns to herbs as their primary medicines. And while drugstore shelves in the United States are stocked mostly with synthetic remedies, in other parts of the world the situation is quite different. For 5.1 billion people worldwide, natural plant-based remedies are used for both acute and chronic health problems, from treating common colds to controlling blood pressure and cholesterol.

Not so long ago, this was true in the United States as well. As recently as the early 1950s, many of the larger pharmaceutical companies still offered a broad variety of plant-based drugs in tablet, liquid, and ointment forms. In fact, the replacement of herbs with synthetic drugs is a relatively new phenomenon, less than a century old, born largely out of economic opportunities afforded by patent laws. Drug companies can't patent plants, but they can develop patented, proprietary synthetic drugs, often reaping billions in sales. Since the 1940s, chemists employed by pharmaceutical companies have developed novel synthetic molecules that have replaced plant medicines and are sold both over the counter and by prescription.

The results of this synthetic drug explosion have been unfortunate. Today, drugs prescribed in hospitals constitute the sixth-highest cause of death among American adults. This exceeds deaths from crack, handguns, and traffic accidents combined. Add to that figure the number of adult and child deaths attributable to over-the-counter and prescription drugs given outside of hospitals, and the figures are even worse. Call me crazy, but I think that this is inexcusable. I believe in the medical maxim "First, do no harm."

I am committed to the development and promotion of plant-based medicines, because they are far and away safer, gentler, and better for human health than synthetic drugs. This is so because human beings have co-evolved with plants over the past few million years. We eat plants, drink their juices, ferment and distill libations from them, and consume them in a thousand forms. Ingredients in plants, from carbohydrates, fats, and protein to vitamins and minerals, are part of our body composition and chemistry. Some compounds perform the same functions in plants that they do in the body. Natural antioxidant phenols in plants, for example, protect plant cells from oxidation, and they often perform the same function in the human body. Our bodies know the substances that occur in plants, and they possess sophisticated mechanisms for metabolizing plant materials.

The same cannot be said about synthetic drugs. These agents are most often alien to the chemistry of the human body, and they're separate and apart from the careful crafting of evolution. Synthetic drugs often act in the body as irritants and toxins, upsetting the balance of whole systems and producing side effects that can be lethal. By contrast, the regular and judicious use of herbs to protect and promote health and as medicines to help treat common ailments is an enlightened approach to personal well-being.

This is not to suggest that plants can't be dangerous. Drink a tea made from oleander leaves or chew a mouthful of foxglove, and you'll be dead in a hurry. On the other hand, if you use any of the thousands of healthful herbs that have been utilized as traditional medicines over the past few millennia, in dosage ranges that have been determined by centuries of trial and error, you are likely to benefit without side effects.

Today we use the term *herbs* to refer to plants or parts of them, including grasses, flowers, berries, seeds, leaves, nuts, stems, stalks, and roots, that are used for their therapeutic and health-enhancing properties. Generations of skilled herbal practitioners, researchers, and scholars have refined and tested the vast science of herbology, producing thousands of plant-based remedies that are safe and effective. The proper and judicious use of herbs is often successful in the treatment of illness when other, more conventional medicines and methods fail. Herbs can be used to cleanse the bowels, open congested sinuses, help mend broken bones, stimulate the brain, increase libido, ease pain, aid digestion, and a thousand other purposes. Topically, herbs can repair damaged skin, soothe a wound, improve the complexion, heal bruises, and relieve aching muscles. Herbs demonstrate great versatility for the treatment of a broad variety of health needs.

In contrast to the dependence on synthetic drugs in the United States today, Native Americans turned to herbs for their medical woes. Two good examples of Native American herbs that provide significant medicinal value are black cohosh and echinacea. Black cohosh (*Cimicifuga racemosa*) has been used for centuries in Native American herbology for the relief of discomfort associated with menopause, and it was listed in the *U.S. Pharmacopoeia* and the *National Formulary*, the two official listings of all drugs that are recognized in the United States. Today, black cohosh is used to relieve hot flashes and other symptoms of menopause. It contains substances known as triterpene glycosides, which directly reduce blood levels of LH, or luteinizing hormone. In menopause, hot flashes coincide with surges of LH. In Germany, many physicians prescribe black cohosh extracts instead of hormone therapy to menopausal and premenopausal women.

Another key plant in Native American folk medicine, echinacea (*Echinacea purpurea* and *angustifolia*) was used topically to treat wounds, burns, infections, and bites. Taken internally, the plant was used as a remedy for stomach complaints, infections, and joint pain. Echinacea has been investigated in more than 350 studies and is considered one of the best immune-stimulating herbs in all of nature. It contains compounds, including echinacosides and caffeic acids, that activate protective killer cells, T-cells, neutrophils, and macrophages in the blood. These agents fight viruses, inhibit infectious yeasts, eat bacteria, engulf tumor cells, and scavenge decayed cells and debris. Echinacea is an herb that helps your body to defend and protect itself.

It is important to note that Native American herbs represent just one group of plants that have significant medical value. Further, health food stores are not the only places where medicinal plant products are found. Rather, plants and plant ingredients from all over the world are widely used in many conventional drugs. *Senna alexandrina*, a shrubby perennial native to Arabia, is just one example of a plant from another tradition that now enjoys worldwide use as a common drug. First introduced to Europe as a laxative by Arab physicians in the 9th century, preparations of the senna plant and its cathartic pods are still widely used today in popular brands of drugstore laxatives. The use of senna has spread as people have learned of its efficacy in moving the bowels. As shown in this case, plant medicines and information about their beneficial effects spread from one culture to another as medicine hunters, doctors, chemists, and researchers discover them and promote their use.

Digitalis purpurea, or purple foxglove, is a popular garden plant cultivated as a source of digitoxin, a cardiac drug that increases the strength of the heartbeat while decreasing its rate. The plant was first recommended for medicinal purposes in Europe during the 17th century, and it has appeared in the French *Pharmacopoeia* since the first printing in 1818. Digitoxin is used worldwide in the treatment of congestive heart failure and other cardiac disorders. In addition, *Digitalis lanata*, or woolly foxglove, is cultivated commercially as a source of digoxin, a cardiotonic used for the same purposes as digitoxin.

Ecuadorian *Cinchona pubescens*, a fast-growing evergreen, as well as other species of cinchona stand among the greatest lifesaving medicines of all time. According to legend, this plant was brought to light in the 1620s when Ecuadorian physician Juan del Vega used a Quichua native remedy then known as quina bark to treat the Countess of Chinchon, wife of the Viceroy of Peru. She had contracted malaria, a potentially fatal disease caused by a protozoan in the stomach of the female Anopheles mosquito. The Countess recovered, and quina bark became known as Countess bark. Word of the cure spread, and in the late 1660s, cinchona was popularized by an apothecary's assistant named Robert Talbor. Over the next 150 years, a huge trade in cinchona bark developed. In the early 19th century, the Dutch established cinchona plantations in Java. In 1820, quinine was isolated from cinchona, and a successful treatment for malaria was established. Today, cinchona is cultivated in several tropical regions, and the approximately 10,000 tons of bark harvested annually yield 500 tons of quinine and the related alkaloids quinidine, cinchonine, and cinchonidine.

Sometimes, the discovery of an herb can be dramatic. Members of Columbus's second trip to the Americas in 1493 were the first non-natives to experience curare—as a poison on the tips of arrows that promptly killed them. On his 1595 voyage up the Orinoco River, Sir Walter Raleigh encountered similar poisoned arrows, launching a legend that spawned the quest to find the source of the poison. In 1799, explorer Baron von Humboldt witnessed a shaman preparing arrow poison from a vine. Von Humboldt brought some of the poison back to Europe, where it stupefied and asphyxiated animals subjected to it. Subsequent explorers attempted to find and identify the plant, but no one could do so until 1938, when an American medicine hunter named Richard Gill found and successfully identified *Chondodendron tomentosum*, the source of curare. This led to the development of the valuable drug tubocurarine, which is used as an adjunct to general anesthetic and in cases of spastic paralysis and plastic muscular rigidity.

Ergot, or *Claviceps purpurea*, is a toxic fungus that grows on grasses and sedges. This unlikely source yields several valuable alkaloids, including ergotamine, which is used to treat migraine. The fungus was recognized as a poison by the Assyrians as far back as 600 B.C., and it was used as a hallucinogen in mystic rites in ancient Greece. In Europe in the Middle Ages, ergot-infected rye flour resulted in mass poisonings, which became known as Saint Anthony's Fire. These poisonings produced delirium, hallucinations, gangrene, and loss of limbs. During the same period, European midwives figured out how to use proper doses of the toxic fungus to induce labor and deliver healthy babies. Interestingly enough, ergot also yields lysergic acid, a derivative of which is LSD (lysergic acid diethylamide). LSD was first made in 1938 by chemist Albert Hofmann in the laboratories of Sandoz Pharmaceuticals in Basel, Switzerland. In 1943, Hofmann accidentally discovered its effects. LSD subsequently became the cornerstone drug of the 1960s psychedelic revolution—and one of the most influential drugs in history.

As is evident from the previous examples, the discovery of beneficial plants happens in a variety of ways. Sometimes medicinal plants are discovered as a result of skilled professional inquiry. But often they're discovered by surprise or even due to sheer serendipity. Through these various means, plants and their derivatives are currently the sources for thousands of drugs worldwide. But this does not mean that these drugs are all safe or free from side effects. Because of their tremendous concentration, some isolated principles from plants, such as morphine, reserpine, digitoxin, vincristine, and vinblastine, are toxic. Whole plants, by contrast, contain hundreds or even thousands of compounds, often synergistic in activity, and are typically safer and often more effective than isolated plant compounds. For this reason, whole herbs and their extracts are undergoing a dramatic increase in popularity as science is corroborating their traditional uses.

Serving as an arbitrary point of demarcation established by drug interests and legislation, the line separating herbs and drugs is becoming increasingly blurry. In European pharmacies, herbs like ginkgo and garlic are often prescribed by physicians, and they've sat side by side on pharmacy shelves with synthetic and plant-derived drugs for many years. The *Commission E Monographs*, a German compendium of herbs, their natural chemical constituents, and their pharmacological effects, is one of the primary references in herbal pharmacy. In the United States, the presence of herbs on drugstore and supermarket shelves is comparatively new. But herbs are gaining popularity quickly, and both pharmacists and physicians are hurrying to better understand them.

We are currently undergoing a renaissance of natural healing and a new era of respect for the healthful treasures that abound in fields, forests, grasslands, mountains, valleys, swamps, and deserts worldwide. But I don't want to paint an overly rosy portrait. The development of natural products, from medicines to foods to textiles, has always been rife with misfits, plunderers, con men, greedy corporate interests, and a plethora of people who don't give a damn about anything but turning a profit. In my research, I run into these types everywhere.

Not everyone recognizes or cares about the importance of the indigenous cultures and traditions of antiquity from which the use of natural, plant-based medicines originates. Nor do many people really care about the environment beyond paying lip service to the notion that it needs to be protected. But real concern for indigenous cultures, traditions of antiquity, and environmental sustainability is required if we are to continue to live on this planet, enjoy natural resources, and benefit from natural medicines. It's our planet. Love it or leave it.

The accounts of my explorations that follow will, I hope, convey valuable information about natural medicine, and will carry you across a threshold to other cultures and traditions. Many indigenous traditions of healing are thousands of years old and reflect a sophisticated appreciation of the wondrous and complex forces of nature. Herbalists, yogis, folk healers, medicine men and women, and shamans possess vast knowledge of medicinal plants and their healing and curative uses, and these people offer valuable lessons about how to live on this precious planet. They typically engage in their plant work with great reverence, and most assume that a higher power guides the workings of the world and all of its living creatures and organisms. This way of engaging in life contrasts sharply with the mechanistic, reductionist, science-as-god attitude that prevails in drug development. The precious value of these people, their cultures, and the natural environments in which they live and from which plant medicines are derived should be evident to all readers. Finally, there is travel upon the trail itself, wild and fantastic, offering up beautiful and exotic places, countless engaging scenes, odd encounters, eccentric characters, and large doses of the unexpected.

Welcome to the medicine trail.

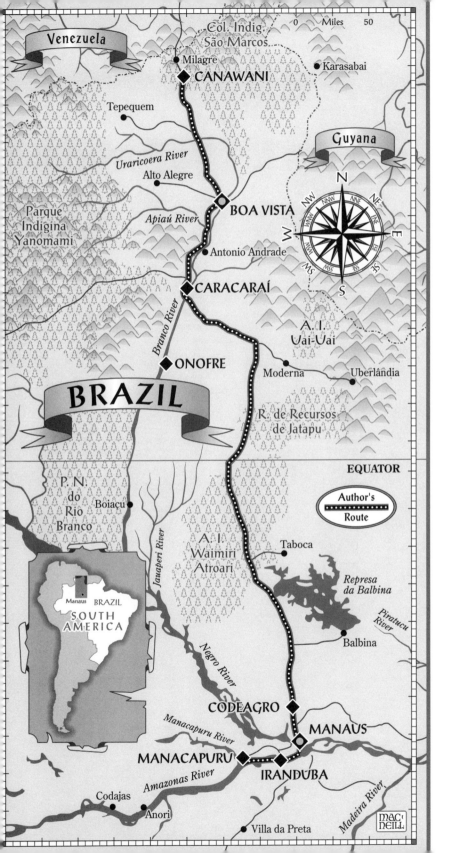

Spirits of the River

THE
SHAMAN'S
DIAGNOSIS

Our jet descended into Manaus, Brazil, through massive gray clouds, beneath which we beheld the vast emerald expanse of the northern Amazon rain forest and the serpentine Amazon river. After collecting our luggage and exchanging money, we waded through a chaotic airport crowd to catch a taxi into the city of Manaus.

This trip was my first to the Amazon, a medicine-hunter's mecca. I had come here to the world's largest river and largest rain forest to meet with native plant experts who know the botanical pharmacopoeia of the region. I sought their guidance for a very specific purpose—to lead me to plant remedies that could be marketed in the United States. I was especially keen to learn everything possible about two legendary sex-enhancing plants—catuaba (*Erythroxylum catuaba*) and muirapuama (*Ptychopetalum olacoides*). My research had indicated that both could be dynamic products in the exploding U.S. dietary supplement market. Now I needed first-hand knowledge.

I was traveling with an Eur Eu Wa Wa Indian by the name of Ipupiara, who was born and raised in the Brazilian Amazon. His Portuguese name is Bernie Peixoto. "Do you know that you can't get a Brazilian passport with an indigenous name?" Bernie asked. "You have to take a Portuguese name or the government won't give you a passport. Can you believe it?" The name Ipupiara, he explained to me, means freshwater dolphin. "When I call out to the dolphins on the river, I call, 'Ipupiara! Ipupiara!' and they come to me. They come right up to the boat."

Bernie's path has not been typical. He underwent years of shamanic training with native elders, earned his Ph.D. in anthropology, and then moved to Washington, D.C. As a shaman, he shuttles back and forth between the daily material world and the spirit world, performing healings, leading vision quests, and seeking information. As an anthropologist, he is an expert on the indigenous peoples from the Pacific Peruvian coast to Brazil's Atlantic coast. And as an indigenous man in the capital of the United States, he has encountered enormous difficulties and endured countless indignities.

When I first met Bernie, he was a guide at the Amazon Exhibit at the National Zoo and a frequent guest speaker in Chelsea Clinton's high school class. He also gave workshops on shamanism and led vision quests. Speaking English, Spanish, Portuguese, and 10 native dialects, Bernie Peixoto is a remarkable tribal storyteller, with a vast knowledge of the environment and cultures of the northern Amazon. When I asked Bernie to go to Brazil with me, he was ecstatic. "Do you know that this is a dream come true for me, to go back and see my people?" he asked me. It would be his first trip home in 10 years, back to his shack where his sister and her family now lived, back to the river and the rain forest. And I couldn't have been traveling with a better man.

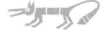

Bernie and I caught a taxi and headed through narrow, busy streets to Mercado Antonio Lisboa. The imposing municipal market, fashioned after Les Halles in Paris, sits on an enviable spot high on the bank of the Rio Negro, the second largest river in the world in terms of volume. Named for its dark waters, which run the color of black coffee, the Rio Negro runs into the Amazon—the largest river in the world—at Manaus.

At the mercado we shopped for hammocks, rice, vegetable oil, manioc, coffee, pasta, and biscuits. We walked through cavernous meat and fish markets with cast iron walls, stained glass windows, and marble counters and purchased a couple of kilos of salted pirarucu, a delicacy fish believed to be the largest species of freshwater fish in the world. "Did you know that these pirarucu are often 2 meters long and weigh over 100 kilos?" Bernie asked, posing his explanation, as usual, in the form of a question. "But so many people catch these, now the fish aren't as big as they used to be." We wandered through crowded aisles of colorful produce stalls piled high with stalks of bananas, oranges, coconuts, hot chilies, onions, greens, tomatoes, fragrant herbs, and exotic local fruits like the viscous-juicy cupuacu and purple acai.

The Mercado Antonio Lisboa bears the markings of the glory days of the Amazon rubber boom, when latex from rubber trees fueled an insatiable world rubber market. From the late 1800s to the 1920s, Manaus was the glamorous, high-society jewel of the Amazon, with French bakeries, Italian stonemasons, and an opulent opera house. The market and the opera house remain, but the bright candle of high society has been extinguished for three quarters of a century. The bottom of the Amazon rubber market fell out when Indonesian plantations produced rubber quicker, cheaper, and in greater volume. Today, Manaus is a crowded, tropical city in the Amazon, with heavy boat traffic, riverside stilt shacks, manufacturing plants of all kinds, and trade zones where popular electronic and other consumer goods are sold cheaply.

The mix of ethnic descents in Manaus includes Portuguese, Chinese, African, and the many different native tribes that live along the Amazon river, in the rain forest, and in the city. In the region we were visiting, members of the Ipixuna, Crinicoru, Macu, Tupi, and Tucano tribes—each with its own language—live interspersed with one another. Interestingly, Bernie was none of these, but rather he is a member of the Eur Eu Wa Wa tribe from the coastal city of Belem, where the Amazon surges into the Atlantic. Bernie, however, had spent much of his life with the Ipixuna outside of Manaus.

At the waterfront, hundreds of boats of all sizes lined the docks. Gangways were packed with passengers and vendors coming and going. Triple-decker riverboats literally packed to the rafters with passengers in hammocks docked side by side with small one-man boats filled with scallions. Laborers toted huge pallets on their heads, piled high with bananas, fish, manioc, cilantro, scallions, and fruit. Most of the men were short, dark, and muscular, and they appeared to carry their burdens with ease. Vendors walked from boat to boat with soda, bread, fruit, cooked meats, and fish. The atmosphere was lively and festive.

Behind the mercado a man named Pedro Roque introduced himself. He had a boat, knew the river well, and would be happy to take us anywhere. We agreed to a price for getting us to Bernie's shack, some 2 hours away. The three of us climbed into Pedro's blue motor launch with our luggage and groceries and headed down the Rio Negro toward its junction with the Amazon, where we would head upriver past the village of Iranduba. The Rio Negro was lined on the bank opposite Manaus by the dense, lush, verdant foliage of the Amazon rain forest. Under muscular gray clouds we sped along the river, stopping at a gas barge to fuel up. A light rain began to fall, and I suggested that maybe it was a poor time to be out on the water. Pedro assured me that in 10 minutes the rain would stop, but he said he'd be happy to take us to the other side of the river—about 12 miles across at that point—to a floating restaurant where we could have some lunch and see whether the sky cleared up. We decided to do that.

As we crossed the great width of the Rio Negro, the rain fell harder and a strong wind blew up. By the time we reached the floating wooden restaurant, visibility had deteriorated and we were battling waves. The rain that Pedro had said would stop in 10 minutes was pelting monsoon-style. "Hey, man, it's really wet, huh?" Bernie commented. I leaped the bow and held us against rising and falling planks as Bernie and Pedro scrambled out. I ran across the planks to the cover of a tin roof and watched rain fall in torrential buckets as the wind howled ferociously. The restaurant was an ingenious floating patchwork of wooden rafts, logs, tin roofing, tables, chairs, tires, and an outhouse perched over the water—all of it anchored in the river. Different sections of the floating eatery were tied together with marine rope, with tires in between. The whole construction chafed and groaned.

As we huddled under the tin roof, I helped to tie down a tarp and a piece of carpet as a makeshift wall to keep out the rain, which was streaming sideways in powerful winds. "I came to a place like this once with some people during a storm," Pedro told us in a nostalgic tone. "It got so bad, the whole house flipped over and broke up, and we wound up in the river for 4 hours. It was very scary, but fortunately nobody died." Bernie and I looked at Pedro and smiled.

As the planks heaved and fell with the swells of the increasingly agitated river, an Indian waitress in a thong bikini continued to work, as did the proprietor, who wore only baggy pants held up by a rope belt. The cocoa-colored old man prepared a feast of succulent fried tambaqui fish filet, rice, beans, macacherra (cooked manioc root), chopped lime, and chilies. Bernie gave me a toothy grin and said, "Welcome to the river, big guy."

When the storm finally broke, we headed off to Bernie's shack, turning from the Rio Negro onto the Amazon. Long islands of dense vegetation, plus reedy grasses and floating flora, filled the river. Pedro, clearly in his element, maneuvered skillfully through the ever-shifting vegetation. Along the way we saw boats small and large, and stilt shacks lining the river banks. Many were submerged up to their windows.

The Brazilian Amazon has two seasons—dry and wet. During the wet season, which lasts for at least 5 months every year, the river rises as much as 20 feet, flooding the ground and forest for miles in all directions. We were at the peak of that season, late May. Water covered as much as two

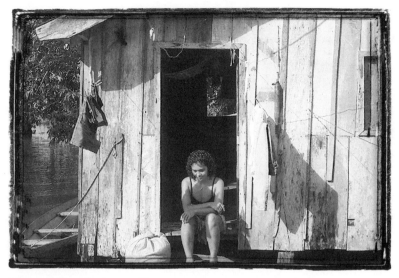

Ipixuna shack on the Amazon River

thirds of the height of some trees, and the borders of the river were pushed back dozens of miles. Only land on hills or raised areas was visible. Great white herons lifted from the grasses as we approached, and bright freshwater dolphin breached from the water. Bernie called out, "Ipupiara! Ipupiara!" A large pink dolphin breached again near Pedro's boat and then rapidly swam away.

After a couple of hours we approached a cluster of shacks, and Bernie announced, "Hey man, we're in my neighborhood." We motored down a long igarape—a water channel cutting through the jungle—to Bernie's place, which was really a small compound consisting of one large tin-roofed wooden shack, one medium-size shack, and a small storage shack. The swollen waters of the river were up to the floorboards of the shacks. Out on a floating pile of logs that served to extend the front porch out into the water, a gnarly dog sat, looking flea-bitten and unhappy. Once we pulled up to the porch, we were greeted by

Bernie's sister María and her husband, José. Also welcoming us were their eldest son Zezinho and his wife Nonata and child Jefferson; another son Passion and his wife Jeriza; a third son Theley and his wife Aldenora; and son Arnaud. All 10 lived together in about 500 square feet of space, and now we were joining them for most of a month. Everyone was especially happy to see Ipupiara—Bernie.

Shortly after we arrived, Zezinho and his brother Passion, both in their early twenties, headed off with Bernie and me in a homemade wooden boat with a 15-horsepower Yamaha engine to get gas for the outboard motor and ice for the fish cooler that occupied a corner of the front porch of the shack. About 10 miles upriver we tied up to a large floating gas barge with a plaza roof just like a drive-up station. Two Crinicoru natives gassed us up. We motored to a floating ice house where a woman scooped huge buckets of chopped ice from a wooden trough into the big Styrofoam cooler on our boat. With that ice, the fish that José and his sons would catch for the next several days would stay fresh.

Back at the shack, I watched two of María and José's sons swim without care in the piranha-filled waters. The image had been implanted in my mind since grade school that a person in the water with piranha is a person stripped clean of flesh within minutes. But, José explained, they normally won't bite unless you're bleeding. This means that menstruating women and people with cuts stay out of the water, but everyone else bathes and swims with impunity. In the dry season, however, when the water is down, some aggressive species, such as the large black piranha, may attack bathers and swimmers.

I was nevertheless circumspect about inserting my body

into the murky depths of the Amazon amidst razor-jawed fish. So I walked along a log that extended out from the back of the shack and began to lower myself into the water slowly enough that I'd be able to pull up quickly if the piranha decided to eat me. Nothing happened. I lowered myself further. All was copacetic. I bathed and shampooed and carried on without a nibble. Later, when I was able to dive right in without being concerned about the piranha, I still remained alert to alligators, anaconda, and poisonous snakes. And I was cautious not to urinate when in the water because of the demonic candiru. A needle-size fish, the candiru (*Vandellia cirrhosa*) swims up the urine stream, enters the urethra, and sinks sharp retrorse spines into the walls of the penis, inflicting a reputedly excruciating pain. Natives, I learned, drink the acidic juice of green fruit of the jagua tree (*Genipa americana*), also known as buitach apple, to dissolve the thin calcium skeleton of the candiru. Otherwise, surgical removal of the fish, and sometimes the glans penis, is required.

After a dinner of fish, rice, pasta, manioc, and broth, Bernie and I got into a boat with the four brothers Theley, Zezinho, Passion, and Arnaud, and Zezinho's young son Jefferson, who was not quite 3 years old. We motored into the dark of night across the river, toward the reeds and grass. Shining our flashlights into the vegetation we spotted the red, luminous eyes of dozens of alligators. Stealing quietly close with our flashlights trained on them, we came right on top of the beasts. Theley leaned over the bow of the boat and snatched three small, angry alligators out of the water. We brought them back to the compound, tied strings around their bellies, and played with them until they were thoroughly annoyed. Then we let them go and went inside.

That first night, Bernie and his family talked by candlelight about the 10 years that had passed since he had moved to the United States. We also spoke about our being there to explore medicinal plants, especially catuaba and muirapuama. At that, everyone broke into smiles. They all knew about the sex-enhancing quality of those barks. Eventually we all retired to our hammocks and swayed off into billows of sleep in the hot, sticky night.

INTO THE FOREST

The next morning at 6:00, María offered coffee in two separate thermoses, both cracked and old. I made a mental note to acquire some new ones for her on the next trip into Manaus. In one thermos the coffee was candy sweet. The other was unsweetened. After coffee, it was time for me to meet the rain forest. José, Bernie, and I climbed into a small canoe and headed across our little finger of the Amazon and into the dense, flooded jungle, filled with bird calls, abuzz with insects, and loud with a million wild sounds. I bailed the leaky boat using half a gourd. It was early in the day, but already the equatorial sun produced sweltering heat. In the mottled light of the forest interior, luminous blue morpho butterflies and brightly colored birds flew in and out of the shadows. Trees held great termite nests and bee hives. Lizards scampered up trunks. A large iguana sunned itself passively on the end of a denuded branch overhead as we glided quietly through the jungle. Far away, like a strange wind, we heard howler monkeys. We were in the land of howler monkeys, but it was hard to get close enough to see them.

The smells of the forest were many—butterscotch, honeysuckle, watermelon, lemon, mildew, moldy bark, meat, feces. We passed through different aroma zones every few feet, one after another, continually. The jungle offered a profusion of floral, carnal, and sometimes indescribable olfactory sensations—some delightful, some almost narcotic, some not so pleasant.

I paid special attention to the thorns. Trees, bushes, and grasses bore them in all sizes. One tree had short, fat spikes. Another was covered with long, hard needles the size of eight-penny nails. Lovely grasses hid evil, needle-sharp thorns on their undersides. Tiny, soft-looking thorns on broad-leafed plants delivered sharp, irritating pricks to the skin. The one thing that these diverse thorns have in common is that they puncture and hurt. We were constantly ducking such armed foliage or carefully pushing it out of the way.

We took on spiders by the dozens as we brushed against branches and leaves. The Amazon is not for the arachnophobic. Tiny spiders no bigger than grains of sand hiked up and down my arms on invisible, filamentous legs. Awkward daddy longlegs walked on spindly appendages over our shirts and hats. Sturdier blue, brown, orange, and gray spiders jumped from branches onto the boat, scrambled over our bodies and faces, climbed up our necks, and then leaped off onto new branches. Some spiders moved slowly. Others responded with astonishing speed as I chased them away from me. Spiders half the size of my hand climbed all over nearby trees.

All the while we were a floating banquet to an endless population of gnats and mosquitoes. Squadrons of vicious-looking wasps flew at us, found nothing of interest, and moved on. In small patches of light, dozens of metallic blue dragonflies hovered in the air, rapidly beating long, delicate, veined wings. Fire ants and black ants large and small came aboard. I gingerly removed a centipede from my shirt with a leaf. I touched the trunk of one slender light gray tree, and instantly more than a hundred fire ants were on my forearm. I plunged my arm into the water up to my elbow and wiped them off quickly. A small praying mantis, a gorgeous green, climbed slowly and awkwardly up the back of José's shirt. Time and again I glanced down at my feet to see a dozen hungry gnats feeding on my flesh. I mashed them all with a single swipe of my hand, repeating the process every minute. As José paddled quietly through the thick, dark jungle, I kept reaching behind me to wipe countless bugs off my back, all the while bailing the canoe.

On the overhanging branch of a tree, José pointed out a large boa constrictor patiently awaiting his next meal. High above in the canopy, nervous, chattering capuchin monkeys leaped from one slender branch to another, dislodging fruit into the water below. When the canoe touched certain leaves, it set off a fluttering explosion of tiny lavender moths, hundreds of them. There were hairy spiders, ticks, chiggers, trees laden with clusters of nasty-looking centipedes. Tiny wasps in groups of several hundred buzzed and hovered around the black, porous bark of one type of tree. Thick clusters of fire ants in piles larger than a fist floated on leaves on the surface of the water, seething and teaming.

"Chris, don't move," Bernie suddenly warned. "Your right shoulder." I turned my head and caught sight of something large and black. Knowing to swipe instead of squash, I brushed what turned out to be an inordinately large black ant off my shirt. "He was going right for your neck," Bernie informed me gravely. "That was a trakwa ant. Very bad. When they bite you, the pain is unbelievable, and you get sick with a fever."

Miles into the dense jungle, we came upon a shirtless Ipixuna in a small canoe. Silently, the man pointed up to a large anteater, easily 40 pounds, making its way slowly along a thick branch. It clawed bark, revealing ants to be hosed up with its long proboscis. I turned to look at Bernie, but he was lost in a deep reverie, back with the spirits of the river for the first time in almost 10 years. The Ipixuna in the other boat gave me a handful of bark. "This is carapanauba," José explained. "We use this for stomach aches and diarrhea." The bark of carapanauba (*Aspidosperma excelsium*), a large tree, is apparently also used to relieve gas and to help control diabetes. I asked the man in the boat to show us carapanauba. We paddled a short distance to a large tree, and I could see where he had cut away some bark.

Later, back at the shack, María and her daughters-in-law Nonata, Aldenora, and Jeriza prepared a large midday meal of fish, rice, pasta, manioc, and bean soup. María wanted to know if the food was acceptable to me. I said, truthfully, that it was fantastic, that I would be happy to eat this way every day, and that no restaurant served fish so fresh and tasty.

After lunch, everybody hit the hammocks. I wrote for a short period, but eventually succumbed to the hypnotic buzzing, chirping, and humming of millions of forest insects. After a brief hammock nap, Bernie, José, and I headed back into the flooded jungle with the intention of catching some pacu, a delicacy fish. When a storm came down upon us, we waited for it to pass under the partial shelter of a huge tree. Continuing through the murky, mysterious floodwaters, Bernie spotted a fat electric eel about 4 feet long right beside the boat. We watched it slither lazily just below the surface.

José paddled the canoe to an acai palm (*Euterpe oleracea*), the small purple fruit of which makes a popular drink in the Amazon. José said that under an acai palm was the place to catch pacu. "Pacu like to eat acai fruit," he explained. "When the small fruits fall in the water, the pacu swim to them. So if you stay quietly in a place like this, you can usually catch pacu." We did see a few, but soon the sky began to rumble loudly. Concerned that it would rain even harder than before, José turned around and headed back across the river to the shack. We had just made it home when the skies opened up and fierce rain beat hammer blows on the tin roof of the shack.

When the rain subsided, Bernie encouraged me to give a water purification demonstration using the portable hand-pump purifier I had brought. The whole family huddled around on the porch as I put one end of a tube into the river and set the other into the top of a thermos-size plastic bottle. As I began to pump water, there were oohs and aahs and a lot of pointing at the purifier as it sucked up river water and deposited it, clean and pure, into the bottle. Little Jefferson wanted to pump water, so I let him have a go. Everyone else would simply drink rainwater, which slid into crockery vessels from grooves in the tin roof, with all the insects and bird crap. I wasn't yet willing to do that. One thing I could control, I figured, was my water intake.

Constant companions inside and outside were the annoying mutuka, which look very much like deer flies. Their behavior consisted of buzzing around us for as long as it took to finally get the opportunity to take a big, stinging bite out of our skin. Sometimes I would sit in the shack and kill mutuka and

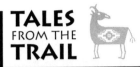
Jungle Unguent

Having to deal with various scrapes, cuts, and bites in the Amazon, I settled on an unguent formula that I found to be highly effective. First, any area to be treated should be cleaned. Then put a dollop of a good herbal salve into your hand. I prefer Herbal Ed's Healing Salve by Herb Pharm, but other salves can be used. Add a few drops each of tea tree, sandalwood, clary sage, and chamomile essential oils. If there is an infection, add some bacitracin or triple antibiotic ointment. Apply this gooey but wonderful concoction liberally. I found it helps to heal most topical problems—including unidentifiable creeping tropical fungal crud—remarkably quickly.

pile them up in a satisfying stack. Bernie quickly found himself with angry, puffy welts all over his body from the unrelenting bites of the mutuka as well as the mosquitoes. I applied essential oils to the welts, and that gave Bernie immediate relief. My bug-bite first-aid for Bernie did not go unnoticed, and soon I had a thriving dermatology clinic going.

I was pleased to be a medicine-bringer as well as a medicine-hunter. I had arrived on the scene fully supplied with a superior armamentarium of natural topical remedies, and the members of José and María's family were grateful for my effective ministrations. José and María both had bites that needed tending, and so I applied oils to those. Then Nonata presented a thumb and an ear that were apparently being eaten away by some kind of jungle rot. I made a gooey concoction of triple antibiotic ointment, Herbal Ed's Healing Salve, and all the essential oils in my kit and slathered the afflicted areas generously. I promised Nonata that I would do this for her at least twice daily, and that by the time Bernie and I headed home, she'd be all fixed up. Little did I know that this simple act of care and kindness would inspire Nonata to cook for me, launder my clothes, and make sure that I wanted for nothing. Little Jefferson, protective of his mother's affections, was not pleased with the amount of time and care I was spending on Nonata's skin wounds. So with a great flourish, I sat Jefferson down and carefully examined and medicated every little bug bite, scrape, and ding on his body with ointments and unguents. He was happy. The clinic was a great success.

We ate an evening meal of fish, rice, and pasta, and then retired to our hammocks for a long, hot night, with all the wooden windows pulled tight to keep the bugs out. Hard, steady rain battered the tin roof. Alligators barked, insects chirped and buzzed. In the middle of the night, a small frog with sticky feet fell onto my chest and startled me awake.

AMAZON DAYS, AMAZON NIGHTS

Before I left Massachusetts for the Amazon, my wife Shahannah told me to be sure to wear protective clothing and the right shoes. But the floorboards of the shack were smooth, the boats were comfortable enough, and more often than not I was standing in water, not on dry land. So I was quickly going shirtless and barefoot, wearing only baggy drawstring shorts. I put on a shirt only when heading into the forest.

Days in the shack usually began around 5:30 or 6:00, with María making coffee. After a long, hot night, everybody in the family would be up, splashing their faces with water either on the front porch or off of the logs out back. Breakfast was typically coffee and some little biscuits, though a few times Nonata made some small pan-fried breads that were delicious. A typical day was more or less without an agenda, stretching wide open before us. "At this time of year with the flooded season, these people don't have that much to do," Bernie explained. "So mostly they catch some fish, maybe repair some fishing nets, and otherwise just wait for the water to go down." Since there's just a very short period in the year to grow onions and manioc and watermelon for market, the subsiding of the water is awaited with eagerness. José faithfully checked the level of the river against small markers on the support poles of the shack at least three times a day, smiling if the water appeared to be a tiny bit lower, and showing concern if it was a little higher.

For the women in the house, the day revolved mostly around food preparation and laundry. The prepared meals of the day, lunch and dinner, usually included rice, manioc, beans, and whatever fish had been caught that day. José, Zezinho, Passion, Arnaud, and Theley all set nets, caught fish with poles, and spear-fished as well. They also ran errands in the boats. Several times Bernie and I went out with the others and set nets along the edges of floating grasses, returning later to retrieve the catch. The waters yielded a great diversity of fish, from large, meaty tambaqui to pacu, catfish, and arawana. The Styrofoam fish cooler on the front porch of the shack usually contained several fish, and occasionally José and his sons would sell fish to other Indians nearby.

Cleaning fish was the task of María, Nonata, Aldenora, and Jeriza, who sat on floating planks behind the shack, vigorously scraping off scales with well-worn knives and throwing fish guts into the water to be promptly devoured by piranha. When fish weren't being cleaned, the women used the same spot for laundry, scrubbing and beating clothes and then hanging them on a line that stretched from the shack to a tree. Nonata attacked laundry with such unrivaled vigor that Bernie and I would receive sparkling clean shirts with smashed and cracked buttons. "That woman is as strong as three men," Bernie said ruefully, examining a spot on one of his shirts where a button used to be. "I would not arm-wrestle that woman. But you gotta admit, this shirt is clean."

Though by no means an expert, José was familiar with many of the local medicinal plants and their uses, and he would point them out to us as we traveled about on the river, canoed in the forest, or walked on higher dry land. Urucum (*Bixa orellana*), also known as annato, is a tall plant with pyramid-shaped seeds. While the plant's fiber is used as cordage and the seeds yield a dye used in foods, the Indians also use a decoction of the leaves for hepatitis, dysentery, and skin problems. The small perpetua-roxa (*Gomphrena globosa*) plant is used for coughs, bronchitis, high blood pressure, and heart troubles. Icao (*Bidens pilosa*) is for dysentery, fever, venereal disease, digestive troubles, and liver disorders. Leaves of the shrub guaco (*Mikania guaco*) are used to treat stomachache, snakebite, and rheumatic pain, and they're applied topically in a poultice to skin rashes. Goiabera (*Psidium guayaba*) leaves and bark are widely used for diarrhea.

The rest of the family introduced me to fruits I'd never eaten before. One afternoon Theley climbed a tree rising out of the flooded yard and shook down inga, long fruit pods that looked like giant green beans and contained a row of succulent seeds coated with a thick, sweet skin. With a long pole, he beat the leaves of another tree, and down came bacuri, which looked like small oranges but contained coated seeds similar to those in inga, but tart. We all scrambled for the inga and the bacuri in the water, as fruit rained copiously and freely from above. María made a drink of acai, which involved grinding the tiny purple fruits of the palm and mixing them with sugar and water. The resulting purple drink was tangy and delicious. On another occasion she and Nonata made a drink of buriti (*Mauritia flexuosa*). The fruits of the buriti palm looked a bit like small pine cones and were hard when picked. But after a day or two of soaking in water, the scaly outsides of the fruit were easily scraped off, revealing a pumpkin-orange starch. María and Nonata mashed the fruits, mixed them with sugar and water, and strained the whole concoction, producing a rich, sweet, creamy drink. Jeriza made a drink of cupuasu (*Theobroma grandofolium*), a sweet, viscous fruit with a floral aroma and a heavenly flavor.

Members of the family taught me enough Ipixuna that I could say a few rudimentary things in their native tongue. *Macca* means I accept. *Ee macca* is no. *Ba* is I, *boa ati* is we, and *ati* is you. *Asu* is big, and *irvi* is thank you. My halting efforts at Ipixuna were a source of entertainment for all, but appreciated.

Every manner of boat traveled up and down the river, from hand-built small craft with 15- or 25-horsepower Yamaha or Suzuki engines to elaborate triple-deckers 80 feet long carrying hundreds of travelers. From José and María's shack we could hear all of the countless motor boats passing by. In the day, we could stand on the floating logs at the back of the house and see the tops of the large river boats above the dense grass that separated the shack from the main body of the river. At night, we heard the churning of engines vibrating through deep waters.

Punctually, just as the sun was setting, the air became thick with bloodthirsty mosquitoes. One moment there were few, and the next moment they were out in full force, attacking face, feet, neck, ears, knees, and thighs with equal zeal. This "mosquito hour" is a phenomenon I've experienced elsewhere in my travels—including India and Central America—but the incomparably aggressive Amazon mosquitoes found body spots usually ignored and left angry, itching welts as evidence of their feasting. Once the mosquitoes arrived, they stayed until sunrise, feeding on any available warm-blooded creature. A quick pee in the middle of the night turned into a riverside bloodsuck. When mosquito hour arrived, we had no choice but to close the screenless wooden windows and doors of the shack and swelter, as many as 12 of us and sometimes more, in the equatorial heat of the Amazon night.

The next morning, Bernie told me that María was going to make tacaca, a very special dish, in our honor. I was all for it, but José warned me that I might not like it. "Don't listen to that grouchy old man," Bernie retorted. "He's just angry because my sister is paying more attention to you and me than to him. Come to think of it, she's paying more attention to you than to me." Bernie then launched into rapid Ipixuna, explaining to María what a horrible guy I was, and why, above all, she should pay more attention to him than to me. María listened with a raised eyebrow. I countered that Bernie was a nasty, duplicitous shaman, not to be trusted. María shook a stern accusing finger at

Bernie, and offered me coffee. "You see that?" Bernie wailed. "Did she offer me any? No. I am fed up with all of you." Then Nonata, my primary dermatology patient, asked if I had any clothes that needed washing. "That does it, man," Bernie seethed. "I'm going to go home and leave you here with these people. You don't need me." Nonata then gave me a big hug, prompting Bernie to throw up his hands and shuffle off to his hammock to sulk. The rest of us fell about the place laughing.

The legend of tacaca is the legend of the Ipixuna, and that's why tacaca is a special dish. When Tupan, the big god, decided to create man and woman, he offered tacaca to the smaller gods and spirits, and to Panema, the dark god. The recipe for tacaca includes a green leafy vegetable called jambu, shrimp, tucupi (the juice of manioc root, which is deadly poison unless cooked thoroughly), a wild onion called sibola, and a sharp-tasting pepper called pimenta de cheiro, or "son of a bitch pepper." According to the legend, pimenta de cheiro was the god Panema's idea. It was his way of adding just a dash of pungent discomfort to the dish.

After offering tacaca to the gods, Tupan asked if any of them knew how to make a flesh-and-blood being in the image of the gods. Yara, the goddess of the water, said, "Yes, I can make all things in my womb, including fish, shrimp, eels, and dolphins." Icorasi, the god of the sun, offered his warmth to the new creation. Jaci, goddess of the moon, said, "I will help the people to grow seeds if they plant them at the proper time." Tupan asked Panema, the god of darkness, what he wanted to offer to the new creation. "I'll try my best to make it hard for this new being to get any crops or fish from the environment," was his reply. "I'll fill their world with bugs, worms, and hostile forces."

Then Tupan said, "Now we have everything we need to populate this land. Cariva (man) will have all this at his disposal. If Cariva shows respect and keeps balance and order, abundance and happiness will be found here." At that moment, Sininga, the god of lightning, and Baraba, the god of thunder, issued forth tremendous lightning and thunder at the same time. The heavens roared. The next day, the first Ipixuna were found floating on the surface of the Amazon.

Making tacaca takes a couple of hours. When María was finished, she called Bernie and me to eat. As we sat at the small table on the porch, Bernie started in again with María. "You know, I don't know why you make such a good dish for this guy," he said to his sister. "I'm an indigenous shaman. I'm the elder here!" His declaration was in vain, eliciting only peals of laughter.

Everybody gathered around to watch my reaction to the tacaca, which was somewhat viscous, a little spicy, and very good. José seemed disappointed that I liked it. Once María saw that I enjoyed the tacaca, she offered me a second bowl. "I can't take this," Bernie moaned. "I'm gonna go throw myself to the piranha."

That afternoon, the house population swelled with the visit of José and María's grown daughters—Sheila, Selye, and Hosannah—and Hosannah's two children, plus a fisherman named Francisco and a medical intern named Cleber. By night-fall, the entire shack was strung with hammocks, each one right next to another. The following morning, after the whole crowd of us survived the uncomfortable night and the roar of Francisco the fisherman's snoring, we were all glad to be up and on the porch drinking coffee. True to my morning ritual, I brushed my teeth, washed my face in the river, and splashed water on my

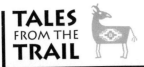

Essential Aid with Essential Oils

Though the natives of the Amazon rain forest know many medicinal plants, not all natives are expert in their use. So all people who explore the Amazon—or any other remote area—would do well to bring with them some natural healing help along with their first-aid kits. The four primary essential oils in the kit I took with me to Brazil possess significant skin-healing properties.

- Tea tree (*Melaleuca alternifolia*) possesses antibacterial, antifungal, and antiviral properties, and thus is a perfect remedy for the various types of tropical crud that plague inhabitants of the Amazon.
- Sandalwood (*Santalum album*) acts as an astringent and enhances the formation of new tissue in cases of cuts, scrapes, sores, and other open wounds.
- Clary sage (*Salvia sclarea*) relieves inflammation and also enhances wound healing.
- Chamomile (*Chamamelum nobile*) is antiseptic and bactericidal, enhancing wound healing and relieving inflammation.

head and shoulders to wake up. There was no room to do any yoga there, but I was content just to squat on some planks and watch the river.

My little medical practice was growing. During early morning dermatology rounds I would examine healing digits, cuts, and dings, and apply essential oils to various new bites acquired during the night. Nonata's ear and thumb were healing beautifully as a result of daily applications of multi-ingredient salve. Hosannah's baby had several bad insect bites, which diminished markedly in size after a couple of applications of essential oils. Her son, who had a scraped knee and an irritated spot under his nose, also improved in 2 days. Nonata's brother Paolo, who also dropped by from upriver, had a small infected gash on his arm, which I treated with ointments and oils. One afternoon María came down with a stomachache and diarrhea, and I made a strong infusion of carapanauba bark, which gave her relief in a few hours. Given that defecating was performed squatting off planks over the water, anything that could reduce the number of times María had to go was helpful.

GERONIMO, THE WILD CRINICORU

"Geronimo's coming," Bernie announced one morning. "He is a good man, except that he is a Crinicoru." It turned out that it was no coincidence that this shirtless man paddling an old canoe toward the shack shared his name with the North American Apache warrior. "The Ipixuna named him Geronimo," Bernie said. "Before tribal warfare was made illegal in the early 1960s, the Ipixuna and the Crinicoru were terrible enemies, and they had grudges that went back for generations. Geronimo killed so many Ipixuna that they gave him that name. He liked it, so ever since he's gone by Geronimo." Bernie pointed at me. "You know how he got his wife? He just came across the river in his canoe and stole her from an Ipixuna village and took her home. Nobody dared to go and get her back. They've been together for a long time."

Geronimo was every bit a wild man. Short and powerfully muscular, with scarred skin like tough leather, he looked as though he had just come out of the swamp, which turned out to be the case. "You know this man almost never wears a shirt," Bernie said. "Even out in the thick jungle, when bugs are biting all over his body. They can't get through his skin." My eyes were

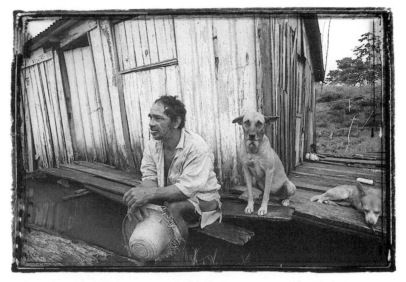

Geronimo, Crinicoru Indian warrior and woodsman

drawn to Geronimo's fingernails, which were more like thick claws, pointed and sharp.

Geronimo explained that he liked to sleep far out in the forest, tied to branches in the upper canopy about 100 feet off the ground. "Don't the animals and insects bother you?" I asked him. Geronimo broke into a wide smile. "No," he said. "They're afraid of me." Bernie teased, "Why don't you like to spend more time with your wife?" Geronimo shrugged, "When I am at home, I want to have sex a lot, but my wife doesn't like to love as much. So I go to the forest." Geronimo spent many of his days and nights alone in the forest, in a canoe, on foot, in trees, in swamps. He fished daily, collected medicinal plants, and observed animals, taking some of them home. "If you want to know this forest, Geronimo is the one," Bernie said. "Even José will tell you that Geronimo knows more about the forest and goes deeper than anybody else." But he also warned that Geronimo tended to get on people's nerves. "This guy does strange things," he said. "He thinks nothing of showing up at somebody's shack at 2:00 in the morning, hooting and knocking on the windows and doors with an oar." Geronimo smiled.

His right eye was missing. There was a time when Geronimo had made a little money by milking cows in the early-morning hours for a man up the river. One night Geronimo tried to quiet an agitated cow by hanging on to her horns, but the strategy backfired when his hands, slick with milk, slipped. The cow jerked its head up, the tip of a horn going deep into Geronimo's eye socket. Geronimo lay on the ground in agonizing pain while the cow, now calm, licked his bleeding socket. After a while, Geronimo stumbled upon some people who loaded him into a canoe and set off in the dark of night for medical help in distant Manaus. But misfortune befell Geronimo a second time that night when a speeding motorboat's wake tipped the canoe. With great effort, Geronimo and the others made it to shore past large, cruising alligators. Finally, as the sun was rising, another motorboat—this one bearing an Indian who'd hacked off a couple of toes with a machete—picked up Geronimo and got him to the hospital in Manaus.

Geronimo offered to take us into the jungle to show us catuaba and muirapuama, both of which grew nearby. "How did you know we wanted to see those?" I asked. Gossip, it seemed, traveled fast along the river. "They all know about us and what we're doing," Bernie said. "We got good publicity. Once we get back from seeing the shamans, we'll go with Geronimo to the forest."

A RIVERBOAT ESCAPADE

I was aware that I could never truly get to know the medicinal plants of the Amazon without learning from those who understand the plants best—the local shamans. These are the individuals who reputedly possess the most developed skills of diagnosis and the greatest knowledge of using plants to heal. More than that, shamans are the keepers of the spiritual flame, acting as intermediaries between the material and spiritual worlds. They are mystics, priests, doctors, and counselors all at the same time. It was a major part of my mission to seek them out.

Aware of my eagerness to visit some shamans in the area, Nonata was able to make the connections for me. Bernie indicated we'd have to rent a boat bigger than any the family had, which we were able to do for $150. The reason for that became clear when I asked how many of us would be going. "Everybody," Bernie replied with a toothy smile and a finger in the air. "Nobody wants to miss this. This will be like a holiday. You just wait."

Early the next morning, as everyone else in the shack slept, I listened as a group of howler monkeys made their way along the trees far upriver. Their howling built to an eerie, primal roar, eventually dying down as they worked their way out of earshot. A short while later, in the mosquito-dark, the entire family was up and preparing to go see shamans up the river. Just as the first dim light of day peeked under the curtain of the horizon, a large, two-decker riverboat named the Zuzimar Filho II docked at the shack. The big Styrofoam ice chest, coffee thermoses, hammocks, luggage, clothing, laundry, bags of food, pots, pans, and two parrots that needed to be fed every day were loaded onto the boat. The hired crew—a sister and two brothers, one in a T-shirt reading "Anaheim Mighty Ducks"—helped us load. "You see their features?" Bernie asked me. "They're Macu. That's another group of Indians who live not too far away from here."

Once we were packed and on the river, we stopped off at the shack of Nonata's brother Paolo, where we took on Paolo's wife Katya and their three children. "Nobody wants to miss this," Bernie chuckled. "Most of these people don't know whether to believe in the shamans anymore. The missionaries come around and tell them that the shamans are the devil, and that Jesus is the only way. The young people know a little about medicinal plants, but they think that drugs in a store are better. They want to be modern, not traditional like their parents or grandparents. So when we want to go see shamans, it makes them very curious."

We motored up the Amazon as the sun rose and light splashed on the water. Greens of all shades and intensity were revealed as trees and shrubs and grasses came to light. The river water turned from black to blue, and the Amazon awoke. On the top deck I took advantage of the dawn to photograph in perfect light. The sun felt warm on my face. Wearing a T-shirt that read "Sailor Man" in stretched letters across her chest, Nonata brought me coffee. In short, all was right with the world.

There was a loud thud. The engine sounded markedly unwell, and the boat began to slow down. The two Macu brothers and the rest of the men trooped off to the engine room, where the floor was soon covered with nuts, bolts, wrenches, and grease. The problem, it was quickly discovered, was that a critical coupling plate on the housing of the driveshaft had broken off. "Hey man," Bernie remarked, "we're worse than up a creek without a paddle. We're up the Amazon drifting backward." It was true. I looked out an engine room window, and we were indeed heading sternforemost downriver. One of the inevitabilities of medicine hunting is that you will have transportation problems.

What ensued was something akin to the Keystone Cops performing boat repair. With much pounding of large hammers, several pieces of hardware were beaten and bent in an effort to fashion a part that would perform the function of the uniquely shaped coupling plate. The Macu captain finally announced his decision to fit two jury-rigged pieces together, which would require sawing the driveshaft in half. Since nobody seemed concerned about this plan that would render the boat inoperable, it fell to me to suggest an alternative—calling for help on the radio. The captain thought this an inspired idea, and the others responded with approving nods. The radio call produced news that a boat would come and take the coupling plate to be welded. "Yeah, man," Bernie said. "They got guys out in the jungle who can weld. You can't believe some of the stuff that's out there."

Meanwhile, we drifted backward down the mighty Amazon. Passion and one of the crew brothers tied a rope to the boat and then to a life preserver, threw the preserver into the water, and leaped in. Holding on to the preserver, they swam toward the grassy river's edge, attempting to pull the boat—a fruitless, Sisyphean task. Finally, a local who'd been watching us from a riverside shack came after us in a small motor boat and towed the Zuzimar Filho II far enough into the grass to stop the drifting. Thus lodged, we waited for help. With little else to do, we set out a bottle of cane alcohol known as caninha, along with lemon and sugar, and started drinking. It was not quite 9:00 A.M. But it was a holiday.

The boat showed up, and a Crinicoru took away the broken coupling plate. Less than 2 hours later, he was back with the welded coupling plate, a bill for $20, and a promised 10-year guarantee on the job, which was dismissed out of hand by all as soon as I paid him and he left. After all, they laughed, that guy is a Crinicoru. We all headed back into the cramped and greasy engine room, and watched as the two crew brothers put the coupling plate back onto the driveshaft with a lot of grunting and grease. Passion and I pitched in when help was needed, and Bernie ran color commentary: "Yes, sir. Here we are in the wild Amazon, where two Macu and an Ipixuna and a gringo are fixing a riverboat. This is the real native experience."

With the coupling plate back on, the captain started the engine. The driveshaft only shook, wobbled, and banged. We'd need to re-seat the entire engine. A job of that magnitude required all hands, plus wooden posts for leverage, ropes, a pulley, and tremendous groaning, sweating, and lifting. About an hour later, we had re-seated the engine, and the driveshaft, though still somewhat wobbly, turned well enough that the captain figured it would last the trip.

We spent the rest of the day chugging up the Amazon, watching birds and boats, and waving at people in shacks by the riverside. Paolo, Nonata's brother, caught up with us in his motorboat, tied it up to the Zuzimar Filho II, and came aboard with his boat in tow. The Macu sister of the crew, who would normally cook for people on the boat, was displaced from her own tiny kitchen by the Ipixuna women of our contingent. The women cooked, cleaned, and did laundry off the back of the boat. Nonata asked if I had any clothes that needed washing, prompting a moan from Bernie. "Sickening," he muttered.

By nightfall the bottle of caninha was empty, we were all fed, and the boat was tied up by a riverside cattle ranch for the night. I was hoping for a cool, bug-free night on the river, but the air was thick with mosquitoes and large, evil-looking night wasps. I snapped my notebook shut on one. The crew sister offered me the top bunk in the tiny forward cabin where she occupied the bottom bunk. Weighing that against the night wasps, I accepted. That prompted Bernie to start in: "You're going to need a very good alibi, sleeping in a tiny little cabin with a single Macu woman. I'm going to tell your wife." In the hot, stifling cabin I languished in a wretched sleep with jumbled dreams.

The next day, we docked the Zuzimar Filho II at a village near Nonata's shamans. Bernie, José, Passion, Paolo, Arnaud, and I climbed into Paolo's motorboat and headed off to see Edna, a woman whose powers of diagnosis were said to be remarkable. We pulled up to a decrepit waterfront shack, where a bony dog lazed on a rundown porch littered with piles of dog crap. A woman appeared at the shack door. Edna was short, with what looked to be a large beer gut. She wore a baseball cap sideways, covering a messy tangle of fiery red hair. A crooked, toothless smile spread wide across her elastic face. Bernie and I went forward; the others hung back, content to be spectators. "We have been looking forward to meeting you," I told Edna. At that she burst into a raucous laugh, contorting her face and shaking her great belly.

Bernie explained to Edna who we were and why we had come to see her. "We have both come a long way, from the United States," Bernie explained. "Yes, but you're from here," Edna said to him. "You are searching for something. Maybe you are trying to regain your power. The years have not been kind to you." Bernie steered the conversation in a different direction. "My friend is interested in the ways that shamans diagnose illness and how they cure with plants," he said. Edna eyed me up and down and nodded. "Do you want me to examine you?" she asked me. It wasn't what I had expected, but, I thought, why not experience what Edna does firsthand?

"People come from all over to see me," Edna said, and then pointed to me. "Some of them come from very, very far, like you." She then mentioned two rules that we would have to agree to. One, we would not try to pay her anything. Two, we would not thank her for anything that would happen there.

Bernie and I looked at each other, shrugged, and agreed to the terms. Edna seemed satisfied that we were sincere. "You know, yesterday, I went to a sacred place to worship the spirits," she said. "They told me that today, two people of good, happy spirit would visit me. I already know from looking at you both that the spirits were right."

Edna, despite her girth, moved with speed. "Have a seat right here," she said, pointing to a small wooden stool in her modest front room. Then she disappeared behind a curtain for a few moments and returned holding a small vassourinha plant (*Scoparia dulcis*), complete with roots. "We call this 'little broom,'" she said. "With this plant, I will know many things about you." While I knew vassourinha is typically used for bronchitis and fevers and to normalize blood sugar in cases of diabetes, Edna apparently intended to use the plant for divination purposes. She began to run the little plant over my face, head, chest, and shoulders, just grazing me with the tip of the tender green leaves. She asked if I had any chest problems. None that I knew of, I answered. "You seem to be in good condition overall," she diagnosed. Then she added, "But several people have put the evil eye on you."

At that moment, I had one of those uh-oh feelings. Bernie and I had traveled to the Amazon at some considerable expense and trouble, and we had hired a riverboat to get to Edna. And there she was, handing me a stock line typical of the lowest-common-denominator Miami psychics. I felt like an idiot. What had I expected, some kind of mystical communication?

But then she said a few things that caught my attention. "There are some people who are putting obstacles in your way and are trying hard to interfere with your work," she said. And she was right. In fact, she was eerily correct about that statement. I listened more closely.

"These people envy your successes," she went on. "And they are very angry because they believe that they deserve what you have achieved by your own hard work. Now they are trying to cause you harm." She went on to describe the specifics of a situation that was causing me some angst. There was no rational explanation for how Edna could have known such a thing. Even Bernie was unaware of the annoying situation I faced in my professional life, in which three disgruntled and incapable individuals were attempting to sabotage my work and reputation. How did she know that?

"If you want to remove these obstacles from your path, you must believe in the protective power of the spirits, and you must also take a bath three Fridays in a row, using two protective plants, mané velho and cheirro cheiroso. These will help you to ward off this evil energy," Edna advised. I told her that I would follow her advice. But, I asked, how did she know about this circumstance in my work life, a world removed from her shack in the Amazon?

"I get knowledge through the plants," she told me. "I must use whole plants with roots, because then the plant is connected to the earth spirits. When I run the plant over your body, the spirits communicate through the plant to tell me what is happening or what is wrong. I get the knowledge in my heart, right here." Edna pointed to the center of her chest and grinned. "After that, a picture comes into my head, very clear, and then I am able to tell you what I see. Do you understand?"

I told Edna that I understood what she was telling me, but that such a thing was not part of my experience. She nodded and threw her hands up into the air, crying, "That's because I am a shaman, and you are not." She burst into a raucous laugh. "But perhaps someday you will be as well. I think maybe so. The spirits are with you."

Edna summoned Bernie to sit on the same stool I had occupied, and she repeated the diagnostic process, touching his face, head, chest, and shoulders with the little broom. When she was done, she looked Bernie in the eyes and nodded slowly. "You are very tired," she said. "The past several years have been difficult for you. You have struggled, and many times you have given up hope. You have lost faith in the spirits, and you have suffered much. You have lost a lot of power." Tears came to Bernie's eyes as he acknowledged that he felt apart from his own world, estranged among people who didn't care for him. "Yes, all of this has hurt you," Edna said, holding a finger in the air. "But I see that slowly, circumstances will begin to change. Coming here is part of that change. You will see. In time, you will regain your power. But you must trust the spirits. Only the spirits can help you reconnect to your world." Edna recommended that Bernie follow the same course of protective baths that she had prescribed to me.

We passed a few hours with Edna, who gave us a couple of handfuls of the mané velho and cheirro cheiroso plants for our baths, and further supplied us with rue (*Ruta graveolens*) and comfrey (*Symphytum officinale*), which she recommended as teas—the rue to further ward off evil influence and the comfrey to strengthen us from within. She was generous and sincerely wanted us to do well in our lives. Did she have an apprentice? "No," Edna replied. "The young people don't want to learn these ways anymore. I have nobody to teach."

I took a few photographs, most of which caught her laughing, and Bernie and I both told her she was a lovely woman, that she had been very kind to us, and that we would never forget her. This pleased Edna greatly, and she enveloped each of us in a warm hug, with plenty of belly. But we did not pay her or thank her. We simply said goodbye and left, wishing her the blessings of the spirits. As we got into Paolo's boat to head off, José asked Bernie and me, "Did you get anything of value from that old lady?" Edna stood on her porch, waving goodbye and smiling her crooked smile. "Oh yeah, man," Bernie said, finger wagging in the air. "That old lady Edna, she knows some things."

NAZARETH'S MEDICINE

The morning sun spilled orange light against the purfled, puffy clouds that stretched across the sky. A large vulture flapped across the river and soared into the forest. By the grass at the river's edge, an alligator slowly sank out of sight. Insects buzzed, fish splashed, and the greens of the forest warmed up and brightened as the morning light increased. Bernie stood beside me on the deck of the Zuzimar Filho II. Today we would see Nazareth, who, Nonata had said, stood out among the local shamans for her expertise in medicinal plants.

At my morning onboard clinic, Nonata presented her greatly improved thumb and ear for examination. Paolo requested topical relief for new bites, and his wife Katya shyly showed me a couple of angry bites on her neck. José had me take a look at a small gash on his thumb. The Macu girl crewmember offered a scrape on her leg for doctoring. Young Jefferson stuck out his bitten arm and belly for diagnosis and treatment. We were a scraped, bug-bitten bunch. I tended to all with various combinations of alcohol swabs, iodine, essential oils, antibiotic ointment, herbal salves, a few well-placed bandages, and assurances of speedy recovery.

After coffee and pan bread, Bernie, Theley, José, Paolo, and I climbed into Paolo's boat and set off to see Nazareth. As we sped along the surface of the water, I reveled in the wind and the fragrant, oxygen-rich air. I thought about the sad fact that at current rates of deforestation, the Amazon would be nothing but a museum exhibit in about 80 years. How, I wondered, could thinking human beings allow such a horrible thing to happen to the most majestic forest in the world?

Like Edna, Nazareth lived by the river, but in a tidy shack that betrayed constant care and attention. We stepped onto a well-kept porch. Nazareth was only 64, but her skin looked weathered beyond her years. Yet her eyes shone with great warmth, and she appeared trim and fit. We introduced ourselves. "I knew to expect you," she stated matter-of-factly, inviting us inside. Colorful throw rugs lay on a spotless floor. Numerous pictures of Christ hung neatly on the walls, and neat Christian statuary sat atop tables and shelves. As is the case in so many other parts of the world, the encroachment of Christianity in the Amazon has resulted in an amalgamation of traditional tribal and Christian beliefs and practices. While some natives consequently eschew their own heritage and native spiritual world view, others simply add Christianity into the mix. Nazareth held firmly to her close affiliation with the spirits of the river and the forest, while simultaneously accepting Christ. For her, this was no contradiction and created no tension.

Nazareth's home was the tidy dwelling of a fastidious woman. Wearing a simple cotton print dress and a silver likeness of the head of Christ around her neck, Nazareth conveyed an aura of peace and contentment. As soon as Bernie mentioned that we were especially interested in medicinal plants, Nazareth flew into high gear. Previously the picture of serenity, she dashed out the door of her shack like a sprinter off the block, returning only moments later with an armload of plants. Speaking rapidly, she proceeded to hand over one plant after another, giving us its name, its use, and any special points. After racing through the entire armload, she dashed out of the shack again.

We followed Nazareth outside and watched her leap off the back of her shack and rush up a slight grassy incline to a large group of plants at the edge of the forest. Bernie whistled in amazement. Like a woman on fire, she dashed around the plants, pulling a leaf from one, a stalk from another, a flower, a bean pod, a fruit. Jumping back onto her porch, she unloaded the plants as before, this time somewhat breathless, as though only the rapid sharing of information would prevent her from exploding. Bernie and I stood laden with unfamiliar plants whose names and uses we couldn't remember, while Nazareth sped off to a cluster of shrubs. We both laughed and clutched our plants. "Maybe," I suggested, "we can get Nazareth to slow down just a bit."

When Nazareth returned from her third forage, we caught her attention long enough to confess that we weren't capable of absorbing such a rapid torrent of information. She looked at us, her fervor visibly diminished. "Oh," she said. Then she invited us back inside to sit down. "Maybe I was a bit quick," she offered thoughtfully.

For the next few hours, Nazareth told us about dozens of plants and described their uses. Some of the plant names she gave were in Portuguese, some in native languages. I subsequently identified many of the plants she described by referencing my notes with botanical books. Several proved to be popular plant remedies used widely by numerous native groups in the Amazon, but not much anywhere else. The few plant remedies that follow hint at the vast pharmacopoeia of medicinal rain forest plants that are still relatively unknown—and unavailable—in the United States but are regularly used by Nazareth and the native people of the Amazon.

❂ Andiroba (*Carapa guianensis*). This is a huge tree, the fruit capsule of which contains oil-bearing seeds. Andiroba seed oil is used as a household liniment to rub on muscle sprains, rashes, sore and inflamed tissue, and skin tumors. It is used to remove ticks and is also applied to the skin in cases of infestation by some types of parasites. Indians use andiroba oil by itself or mixed with annato oil (*Bixa orellana*) to repel insects. The bark of the andiroba tree is made into an infusion for internal use in cases of fever and intestinal worms. Nazareth explained that making infusions of tree barks was commonly accomplished by placing a small handful of bark in a vessel of room temperature water, letting it sit overnight, and drinking the resulting liquid in the morning.

❂ Aripari (*Macrolobium acaciaefolium*). This tree's wood is commonly used for making boats, but the bark of aripari is taken internally as an infusion to relieve diarrhea. Topically, finely powdered leaves are used to treat ulcerated wounds.

❂ Mastruco (*Chenopodium ambrosoides*). This common tropical plant is astringent and highly aromatic. Dubbed "wormseed," mastruco contains ascaridole, a nematocide that kills ascaris, a nematode parasitic in the large intestine, and oxyrus, a large species of pinworm. Infusions of the plant are used to kill roundworms, tapeworms, and hookworms and to cure dysentery. An infusion of the leaves is used to relieve flatulence and asthma and to improve breathing. Some native women use mastruco to relieve cramps and as a contraceptive, and the plant is also employed to induce labor.

❂ Quebra pedra (*Phyllanthus niruri*). A leafy shrub, quebra pedra, also known as shatter stone, makes a bitter-tasting tea used as a diuretic, to treat kidney infections, and to eliminate kidney stones and gallstones. Quebra pedra inhibits the hepatitis B virus, and it's under investigation for use in cases of hepatitis and other liver diseases. The plant contains anticarcinogenic agents and is rich in antioxidant phenols, which inhibit cellular aging.

❂ Jurubeba (*Solanum paniculatum*). A popular hangover remedy, jurubeba is used widely throughout Brazil. It's drunk as a tea to relieve discomfort associated with excessive consumption of food or alcohol. Jurubeba tea and extract reputedly work quickly to relieve indigestion and reduce inflammation of the liver and spleen. The plant contains alkaloids and a steroid saponin compound named paniculidin, which may account for jurubeba's liver-protective properties. The leaves, roots, and fruit of the plant are all used.

❂ Tayuya (*Cayaponia tayuya*). A widely used analgesic, tayuya contains cancer-inhibiting compounds known as cucurbitacins, which may additionally inhibit the Epstein-Barr virus. The plant reportedly relieves many types of pain, especially nerve pain, headaches, and backaches. Tayuya is also taken as a general tonic, to regulate metabolism, to cleanse the blood, and to reduce swelling.

The Amazon's Sex-Enhancing Plants: Do They Work?

The libido-lifting and sexual stamina–enhancing qualities of the Brazilian tree barks catuaba and muirapuama are so well-known and widely used in the Amazon rain forest that their legitimacy is seldom questioned there. But the science on catuaba and muirapuama is still thin, though encouraging. Many reports in scientific journals and at conferences have confirmed their sex-enhancing properties and have broadened interest in their use. For example, in one study using muirapuama, 51 percent of men with erectile problems reported improvement, and 62 percent experienced an increase in libido.

A group of alkaloids in catuaba known as catuabine A, B, and C are believed to enhance sexual function by stimulating the nervous system. In muirapuama, chemists have identified a group of sterols, including beta-sitosterol, thought to be responsible for the herb's aphrodisiac effects.

With her own cultivated medicinal garden plots and the great rain forest only steps away from her shack, Nazareth had access to hundreds of medicinal plants that she knew how to identify, prepare, and use. "My father was a great shaman, the best around," she told me. "He knew all about plants, and he taught me different medicines, what they are for, and how to use them. I studied with him for many, many years, and then I knew how to treat people. Now so many people come to me. By the grace of God, I can help them." Did she have an apprentice? "No," she replied sadly, echoing Edna. "The young no longer care about the traditional medicine."

I asked Nazareth if she recommended any specific plants for sex enhancement. "Many people come to me for this reason," she smiled. "Especially men who are having problems. Some-times they have not had sex in years. Nothing works as well as catuaba and muirapuama. They are good for women as well. Taken together every day, catuaba and muirapuama can make people sexually young again."

As the river began to gray in dwindling light, we said goodbye to Nazareth. "You come back here," she said to me. "Come spend several days next time. You will take some sacred plants for visions, and then I will teach you about the plants." I promised to return, and Bernie and I climbed into the boat with the others, who had waited patiently for us the entire day. "Do you believe in those plants?" Theley asked me with genuine curiosity. "That they work?" I looked at him. "Yes, Theley, I absolutely do." As we pulled away in Paolo's boat and headed back upriver to the Zuzimar Filho II, Nazareth stood on her front porch with an armload of medicinal plants, waving goodbye with her free hand.

CAXIRI

Bernie the shaman pushed his chest out, beamed a cockeyed smile, and announced, "I'm going to save you money, big guy." I eyed him warily. Opening his hands with a generous flourish, he continued, "We gonna take the bus to Boa Vista. It's really cheap." I frowned and said, "Are you nuts, Bernie? The bus is cheap because it's a last resort. Do you really want to ride on these roads almost all the way to Venezuela?" He put on his best hurt expression, the one he uses when I challenge his ideas. "Hey man, don't talk to me like that," he said. "I'm your brother."

We were bug-bitten from head to toe and weary from our uncomfortable weeks on the Amazon River. I welcomed the idea of saving money, but the choice between an hour plane flight from Manaus to Boa Vista and a 15-hour overnight bus ride seemed no choice at all. "Let's just fly up there," I tried again. Bernie stuck out his lower teeth in defiance. "Okay, mister big-shot medicine hunter, you go fly and spend lots of money," he shot back. "I'm taking the bus." Of course, Bernie ended up getting his way, since I wasn't about to let him take that bus ride alone, and he knew it. After I gave in, he said with a smug, triumphant smile, "We gonna have a very nice bus ride."

I was traveling to Boa Vista to meet with Gilberto Macuxi, big chief of the Macuxi Indians, one of the primary tribes in northern Brazil. Gilberto was planning a multi-tribal gathering for the following year that would bring together shamans from all over the Amazon. If the gathering worked out, it would be the largest assembly ever of indigenous native healers, and it would represent an unprecedented opportunity to gather valuable knowledge about plant medicines and their uses.

The lurching bus ride from Manaus straight north through the dark heart of the Amazon was anything but "very nice." The paved road out of Manaus quickly became a slick dirt track, with deep ruts, huge puddles, and sections that were almost totally washed out by the heavy rains that batter the jungle. Our seats were right up front, affording us a horrifyingly clear view of the rusting carcasses of trucks and buses that had slid off the soft shoulders of the road and lay half sunk in viper-infested swamps, the sudden swerving turns that seemed to come out of nowhere, and the roaring, heaving trucks and buses that occasionally barreled toward us like phantoms from some mechanical hell. Panicked chickens in baskets clucked in loud alarm as the bus fishtailed on greasy mud. As we bounced and jolted and woozy passengers puked out the windows, I commented to Bernie what a lovely idea it was to take the bus.

Neither Bernie nor I slept a wink. Instead, we stared saucer-eyed at the gloom of the night before us, as the piercing gray beams of the headlights stabbed through patchy fog and illuminated endless miles of high trees surrounded by swamp and hanging with thick tangles of vines. As if he had gone berserk, the driver hammered the bus furiously as though we were in a stock car race. We careened wildly through the dark. There were two stops at roadside stands, where Bernie and I could take refreshment in the form of Nescafé and crackers, and the motion sickness victims had a chance to rinse their vomit-covered shirts and pants at standing pipes. "You like the ride, man?" Bernie inquired at the first stop, near the town of Carimau, right on the equator. I only growled. "You know," he said in a patronizing tone, "bad attitude can make you sick."

We arrived in Boa Vista jittery, sleep-deprived, and covered with slick, pungent perspiration from a night of fear. As we stepped off the bus, I told Bernie, "You can ride this heap all the way back to Manaus if you want, but I'm flying." Bernie winced.

THE DANGERS OF BOA VISTA

The last outpost in the northern Brazilian Amazon, Boa Vista is the only urban area in sprawling Roraima, the northernmost state of Brazil. Billed as a "planned city," Boa Vista is a cattle and petroleum town with a Wild West atmosphere. It's home to traffickers of all kinds who find the location advantageous for moving goods across the nearby Venezuelan border.

We were supposed to meet Gilberto at the bus station, having sent a message to him through some people at Roraima University. "I don't see him, man," Bernie said as we waded through the crowd at the station. Then a handsome Indian with long hair approached us. He wore a crisply pressed sleeveless white shirt, new blue jeans, a braided leather belt, and smart black leather shoes. "Bernie?" he asked. It was Gilberto. The two embraced, and Bernie introduced me to Gilberto, who in turn introduced both of us to a friendly looking man named Domingo. This man had a wrestler's body and a laborer's hands, and he was sweating so profusely it appeared as though he had just showered and thrown on his clothes without drying off. Domingo, Gilberto told us, would drive us around during our stay.

As we walked to Domingo's car, Bernie quietly confided, "I didn't even recognize Gilberto. Last time I saw him, he looked like a truly wild tribal man, with paint on his face and a spear in his hand. I wonder what happened." What had happened to Gilberto is what has happened to many natives of the Amazon. He was slowly and steadily being eaten up by modern culture, losing his tribal identity in the face of steadily encroaching modern society. Nonetheless, he remains a legend in Roraima. Gilberto is a tireless crusader for native rights, part Che Guevara and part Chico Mendes, the martyred Brazilian environmentalist and union leader. He has been jailed and beaten, and has had his life threatened many times for his work defending and pro-tecting tribal people and their lands. Gilberto has traveled to the United States three times, and to Europe four times, to tell the story of indigenous people and to petition for support for their protection and preservation. He wages the same war that many tribal leaders around the world fight against overwhelming odds, against military forces too powerful to defeat, and against huge corporations too rich to stop. It is a losing game.

In Domingo's battered Toyota Corolla wagon, we bounced along the rutted dirt roads of Boa Vista, enveloping pedestrians in clouds of dirt. Honking trucks spewing black diesel smoke, bald-tired cars without mufflers, and Japanese rice-rockets that sounded like popcorn makers charged together down the broader avenues of town, past thousands of almost identical tin-roofed huts. I sat behind Domingo, watching sweat stream down the back of his neck as we made our way through the city's gouged, chaotic streets to the Hotel Euzebio, where Bernie and

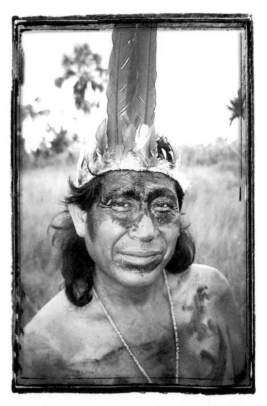

Gilberto Macuxi of Boa Vista, supreme chief of the Macuxi Indians and a tireless crusader for native rights

I planned to stay for about a week. From there we would travel with Gilberto and Domingo to various Indian villages and gather information on regional medicinal plants.

In the hotel lobby, two shifty-looking characters sat stiffly with leather briefcases clutched too tightly to their chests. One had a conspicuous bulge under the left arm of his sharkskin sport jacket, a garment wholly out of place in the sweltering heat of Boa Vista. Standing at the registration desk, a greasy-haired man openly sported a .357 magnum with mother-of-pearl grips in an intricately tooled leather holster on his hip. He looked like a Tijuana loan shark, with a pencil moustache, cruel eyes, and a nasty pink scar that creased the length of one cheek.

The two-story Hotel Euzebio was less a place of lodging than a bustling center of commerce. Most of the guest rooms served as small, inexpensive stores for moving goods and services, from clothing and kitchen gadgets to airplane rides for drug dealers. Dozens of people loitered in the halls. Whether you were after a few inexpensive shirts or a hooker by the hour, the Euzebio was the place to find it. But our room—a small, monastic cell with two narrow single beds—was spotlessly clean. And it included not only a toilet but also a shower with hot and cold running water. As a respite between stays on the river, the Euzebio felt like the Ritz Carlton. I slept like the dead and made up the rest I'd missed during our cost-cutting bus rampage through the steaming, savage jungle.

Gilberto and Domingo came by the next morning and offered to take Bernie and me about 100 kilometers north to an Indian settlement called Canawani. Gilberto was the most freshly pressed man in sight, as though he had just finished a casual native fashion photo shoot for GQ. By contrast, beaming, friendly Domingo had his shirt unbuttoned to hairy midbelly, and he was soaked with sweat. We climbed into the dusty old Toyota that seemed held together with bailing wire and bubble gum, and headed off for the native village.

About 20 kilometers out of town, Domingo pulled over to the side of the road and had me follow him to a tall, leafy tree. It was my first actual look at a jatobá tree, which I knew only from reading and by its botanical name, *Hymenaea courbaril*.

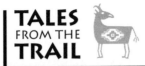

TALES FROM THE TRAIL

A Brazilian Bark with Bite

The inner bark of the jatobá tree, which grows from Brazil up through Central America, is used in the Amazon rain forest as a folk remedy for cystitis, bladder infections, cough, fever, and much else. But jatobá is also reputedly an energy enhancer, and it's sold in the United States for that purpose, usually as a tea.

Here's a way Brazilians like to prepare jatobá for general vitality: Place a small handful of the cut bark in a glass of room-temperature water and let it stand overnight. In the morning, strain out the bark and drink the water. Natives say that this will boost strength and prevent fatigue.

Domingo produced a well-worn jackknife from his pocket and pried off a chunk of bark with a sure, practiced motion. "You boil this in water and drink the tea," he said. "It gives you energy. If you have to work all day, you take some jatobá tea with you, and the work will be much easier. When I worked on my father's cattle ranch, I would drink this all the time." Domingo also lauded jatobá's effectiveness for "many women's problems." Some people, he said, boil the bark and drink the liquid to stop diarrhea. Then Domingo squatted down and employed the knife again to dig a small clump of semi-hard gum from the base of the tree. "In the churches they use this to make incense," he explained. "But this is also very good medicine. You rub it on aches and pains." He took my hand, rubbed a little bit of the sticky material on my wrist, and invited me to smell it. The resinous aroma was infused with terpenes and reminded me of other natural gums that are also used as medicines.

Tree gums, or resins, have been employed as medicines for centuries. Tragacanth gum, from the thorny western Asian desert bush *Astragalus gummifer,* has been used as a stabilizer and thickener in natural medicines since the time of the early Greeks. The oleo gum resin frankincense comes from the trunk of *Boswellia carterii,* a shrub indigenous to northeast Africa and Arabia. One of the most revered of all fragrances, frankincense has been used since antiquity as a ceremonial incense in India and China as well as in Catholic churches worldwide. This is fitting, because frankincense conveys an aroma that quells anxiety, abates nervous tension, and eases the mind. In traditional medicine, the gum is used in topical preparations for wounds, scars, and blemishes. Frankincense holds a unique place in religious tradition as one of the gifts presented by the three wise men to the infant Jesus. A second of those rare gifts, the gum myrrh, comes from various species of *Commifora,* shrubs that grow throughout Ethiopia, Somalia, and Yemen. First mentioned in medicinal texts more than 3,500 years ago, myrrh was an essential ingredient in the Egyptian embalming process and is well-established in traditional Chinese medicine. Myrrh gum is used for cuts, wounds, sores, ulcers, hemorrhoids, inflamed gums, sore throat, coughs, and colds.

FRANCISCA'S BREW

After almost 2 hours of banging, bouncing, dodging potholes, and eating road dust, we arrived in the village of Canawani and saw no one. "I think everybody is out working in the fields," Gilberto commented. We walked through the village until we finally spotted a slender, long-legged man leaning against a supporting post of a small maloca, a hut with a thatched roof. The man introduced himself as Adir and informed us that since the village chief was away, proper etiquette dictated that we pay a visit to Francisca, one of the head women of the village. He offered to come along and make introductions. We crowded back into the Toyota, this time with leggy Adir to fit in, and bounced down the dusty road to the other side of the village.

Francisca owned two malocas, one with walls and one without. The one without walls was apparently the site of heavy food production. The centerpiece was a round, 4-foot-high wood-fired oven topped with a flat-bottomed iron pan about 4 feet in diameter. Called a fugao, this apparatus is used for roasting manioc meal, the grainy flour made from the staple manioc root.

We had, of course, seen—and eaten—much manioc in Brazil. Also known as cassava, manioc (*Manihot esculenta*) has tubers for roots that resemble sweet potatoes in appearance and are prepared to yield a granular, carbohydrate-rich staple food that appears on virtually every Brazilian table. When the Portuguese arrived in Brazil in the early 1500s, they found that the main staple of the native people was manioc. The plant, they discovered, was relatively easy to cultivate, but processing the raw roots into the carbohydrate-rich end product required serious labor.

Manioc root contains prussic acid, a potentially lethal toxin. Poisonous when raw, manioc root must be pressed and cooked in an elaborate and time-consuming process to dispel the prussic acid. The tubers are first peeled and then grated, after which the pulp is prepared by one of two methods. Typically, the pulp is packed into long cylinders called tipitis, which are made of woven plant fibers. Once a tipiti is filled with manioc pulp, it is hung from a house rafter and either twisted by hand or attached to a heavy weight at the bottom end. This compresses the pulp and squeezes out the poisonous juice. In the other method, the manioc pulp is put into a cloth sack that is fitted at the bottom of a heavy press made of logs. Resembling a medieval catapult in design, the press has a long, heavy pole that is pulled down at the far end and tied. The pressure exerted by the press expels the juice from the pulp.

Once the pulp is pressed, it is removed from either the tipiti or the press and placed into a fugao. A wood fire underneath heats the bottom of the iron pan to a scorching temperature. The manioc pulp is placed in heaps upon the hot fugao and then stirred with a large wooden paddle for a long time until it turns into dry granules of coarse meal or flour known as farinha de manioca.

The toxic juice of manioc is collected and left to sit and separate. Starch settles out from the extracted juice. The liquid is poured off, and the starch is placed onto the hot, flat surface of the fugao, eventually clumping together into small, round granules called tapioca. The juice, now free of starch, is cooked, resulting in a nontoxic and delicious condiment known as tucupi, which is often spiked with hot chilies and poured liberally onto meats, fish, grains, beans, and vegetables.

Francisca's fugao was not being used when we arrived; instead, it was piled high with dried leafy branches of the common cayupa tree. I would soon find out why. There were also pieces of beiju, a hard, flat bread less than an inch thick, made of crunchy manioc flour. Francisca welcomed us warmly, shaking our hands with arthritic, sausage fingers. A short, rotund, mostly toothless old woman in a thin, stained smock, Francisca was a native who had been made both strong and old by decades of hard labor. In honor of our coming, Francisca announced with a flourish that she would offer us the ultimate in regional native hospitality—freshly made caxiri (pronounced "cash-er-EE"). This news incited genuine jubilance among Domingo, Adir, and Gilberto. Bernie, I thought, appeared more circumspect. I didn't yet understand what was about to transpire.

I am far from squeamish. I have eaten cooked insects without complaint, and I accept virtually all dishes offered to me in far-flung corners of the world, where ingredients are unfamiliar and hygiene questionable. But what ensued was one of the most horrifying food-related scenes I have ever witnessed. I could hardly believe my eyes when from under a table Francisca dragged a large metal pot, brimming with a foaming yellowish substance that looked very much like vomit and was aswarm with flies. Setting the pot down, she picked up a red rubber washbasin filled with soiled laundry soaking in milky gray water and emptied it on the ground. Pouring a small amount of fresh water into the tub, she swished it around with a brief circular motion of her short, thick arms, and emptied it. That brief rinse accomplished, Francisca was ready to make caxiri.

Pointing proudly at the pot, Francisca explained that she had carefully chewed and spat cayupa leaves and manioc flour into the vessel for 3 weeks, and that the whole batch had been fermenting for 4 months. "Oh, God," I thought as I realized I would be offered a beverage made from the insalivated muck that bubbled before me. I thought of the fly excrement that had been incorporated into the ingredients, and envisioned a host of pathogenic bacteria invading my entire body and setting up shop. Francisca announced with great gusto that caxiri is the best of all foods, a drink so potent in its health-imbuing power that after consuming it, one can toil tirelessly in the fields all day long. I turned to Bernie with wide, pleading eyes. "This is the real indigenous stuff," he said, his magnified eyes narrowing behind the thick lenses of his glasses. "You're really going to love this delicious, hygienic drink."

Francisca laid a woven-fiber straining mat framed by wooden sticks over the washbasin. Then, employing both hands, she scooped up a pile of the bubbling mixture and plopped it onto the mat. She poured some water from a small crock over the mound and proceeded to knead the mixture vigorously with her thick fingers. As she worked the mess, liquid trickled steadily through the mat into the washbasin. I felt a crawling sensation along the hairs on the back of my neck. Bernie smiled wickedly, relishing the moment. Now Francisca was up to her stout elbows in bubbling caxiri, waxing effusive about its manifold health benefits. "It is the very best for the stomach," she said. Bernie nudged me. "You hear that, big guy?" he asked. "It's good for your stomach." I told him my stomach was fine. Francisca, just warming up, then let us know that caxiri was good if you're having trouble with your urine. Bernie smiled at me again. "My urine is perfect," I reported. "Get us out of this, whatever you have to do."

I was aware of fermented manioc beverages made by insalivation. The Maya make a drink they call balche, into which they sometimes add hallucinogenic plants for an extra kick. Peruvians commonly drink chicha, which is also made by chewing and spitting manioc. But in both cases, the drinks are complete within a couple of days. And while there is no question that you could still contract hepatitis or a pathogenic bacteria from either balche or chicha, they seemed to me drinks that you could more easily survive than Francisca's caxiri, which had been stewing for 4 months in fly shit. On the bright side, a fermentation period that long would render a high alcohol content, which just might kill anything in the drink. But I still wasn't eager to find out.

By this time, Francisca had practically burst into full-throated operatic song, extolling the manifold virtues of caxiri. And God bless Francisca, for she was performing hard labor on our behalf, to make for us the thing she prized most. Her intentions were golden, her spirit generous. Gilberto, Domingo, and Adir appeared as excited as school boys at a ball park as she heaped more yellowish muck upon the mat, wetting and kneading it, and squeezing the evil, septic drippings into the poorly rinsed laundry basin. Pursing his lips and nodding

Francisca making caxiri, a beverage of fermented manioc root

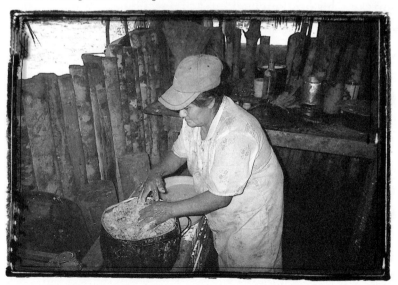

thoughtfully, Bernie once again expressed his considered opinion that it would be good for me to have this "real indigenous experience." I resorted to bargaining. "Okay," I told him. "You drink and I'll drink. Whatever you do, I'll follow." Bernie backed up a step and held up his video camera. "I'm just a cameraman," he said. "You drink and I'll shoot, all right?" I held my ground. "No deal, Bernie. You drink and I'll drink. We'll die together."

The moment of reckoning was upon us. Francisca filled a tall steel cup for each of us, and we all made toasting gestures. I felt like a condemned man taking a last drink before execution. I raised the cup to my lips, noticing a pleasant banana aroma. "Don't drink that," Bernie said under his breath. "Give me yours and take mine." I did as instructed and received an empty cup for my full one. I gave Bernie a sidelong glance and asked him secretly if he'd drunk his. He shook his head. With Bernie's sleight of hand, we both wound up with empty cups and were spared. Domingo, on the other hand, went on to consume four, smacking his lips loudly after each one. Gilberto and Adir had two each and proclaimed that Francisca's was some of the best caxiri they'd ever drunk. Bernie and I respectfully declined seconds, slapping our bellies and declaring that the first tall cup had filled us up.

I had mixed feelings about my reprieve. On the one hand, I was truly appreciative of Francisca's kindness and generosity. But realistically, I was relieved to avoid drinking a brew that might have debilitated me with dysentery or hepatitis. Francisca picked up an aluminum pot and pointed to numerous small holes around the bottom. "If you leave caxiri overnight in a pot like this, it makes these tiny holes, see?" With that information, I was no longer conflicted about my decision.

We all expressed our gratitude for Francisca's hospitality, and we enjoyed a little beiju, the hard and mildly sweet manioc bread. Domingo proudly stowed a jug of caxiri that Francisca had given him in the hatchback of the Toyota. After goodbyes and handshakes, we piled back into the car. As we drove down a dusty dirt road, I could hear the bubbling caxiri gurgling and fizzing underneath the cap.

A MEETING OF NATIVE CHIEFS

After spending a little time in Canawani, we said our goodbyes to Adir and rumbled back toward Boa Vista, to a meeting of tribal chiefs at the small headquarters of APIR, the Portuguese acronym of a grassroots organization that helps sick, homeless, or destitute native people. "In a lot of cases, Indians just come wandering in out of the jungle," Gilberto said. "Sometimes they are very sick, or hurt, or totally messed up from hunger or because they have been abused. At APIR they can get some rest and a little medical help if they need it, and also they can get food." The halls of the concrete APIR headquarters were stacked with plastic bags filled with grains, sugar, and other staples—all to be given away to Indians being run out of the forest with no place to go. "It is not enough," Gilberto said, gesturing at the care packages with a wide open hand. "It is never enough."

Inside a shabby room that served as the APIR office, Raymundo, a chief of the Macuxi Indians, sat behind a beat-up metal desk on an ancient swivel chair, while others sat on rusted metal folding chairs or on the floor. In Brazil, tribes of size typically have many chiefs of varying ranks, in the same way that an army may have numerous generals from one-star to four-star.

Gilberto was supreme chief of the Macuxi, but Raymundo was of high rank and very highly regarded. Here he was chairing a meeting to discuss the gathering of tribes planned for the following year.

Periodically, Bernie leaned over and translated bits of the discussion, which was conducted in Macuxi: "They say that they want to have this very important gathering on sacred land, but that the government agencies are doing everything they can to prevent the gathering. They say that government officials are pretending to be helpful, but are demanding all kinds of licenses and papers that these people don't know how to get. You watch, this gathering they want to have will be very difficult to make happen."

After the somber meeting, I was waiting outside in the shade when Chief Raymundo emerged from the APIR building wearing a feathered headdress and carrying a hunting bow and a long blowgun. He was also sporting a T-shirt with an incongruous cartoon bear on it. The ever-energetic Domingo picked a small leaf about the size of a finger from a bush and pressed it against the bark of a tree at about head height, making the leaf stick. He took the 7-foot-long hardwood blowgun from Raymundo, hefted it to shooting position, took a large breath, and blew off a shot. He missed the target by a foot or more.

Miguel, a dark-haired man with a handsome face and a quiet manner who also carries the title of chief, motioned for the blowgun from Domingo, as if to show him how to do it right. Miguel slid a long wooden dart into the mouth end of the blowgun, feathered the back end of the dart so it fit the blow hole just right, lifted and sighted the blowgun, and missed hitting the leaf by a few inches. The misses of Domingo and Miguel prompted a round of shots on the part of about 10 Indians. One by one they tried, none getting near the leaf. Several missed the tree entirely. Only Miguel hit close.

I asked if I could take a turn, hoping it wasn't a breach of protocol. They were happy to let me try. I fitted the dart into the blow hole, feathered the cotton end to fit just right, and hefted the heavy wooden shaft. The leaf was about 25 paces away. I recalled the basics of shooting from when I was a teenage crack shot with a .22 caliber rifle. The principles were the same. Aim, steady, fire. I took a large breath and, with as much compression as possible, blew the dart out with a punch, missing the leaf by only an inch or so. This provoked some murmuring from the Indians. Beginner's luck.

Several more Indians tried again, but the only one who shot close was Chief Miguel. He also missed by about an inch. I put myself in the rotation of shooters, and missed again by only about a finger's width. Miguel shot again and came close, but didn't hit the leaf. The others gave up shooting, and that left Miguel and me to pass the blowgun from one to the other while the Indians divided into two groups—one standing beside Miguel, the other beside me, like cheering sections. Jurcelina, Gilberto's daughter, declared that this was the international blowgun contest between the indigenous Indians and the United States. The pressure was definitely on.

As Miguel and I each shot and missed by incredibly tight margins, our teams applauded and shouted: "Come on, hit the leaf." "Go U.S. You can win." "Miguel, you have to beat him for all the Indians." Miguel and I were both aware of the silliness of the situation, but neither of us would give up. We were in this contest until one of us hit the leaf.

After about 30 turns each, the right thing happened. Miguel hit the leaf dead on. Everybody cheered, and I shook his hand and congratulated him heartily. We both laughed, and each of us wiped sweat from our foreheads. Chief Miguel gave me a look that seemed a mixture of relief, respect, and friendship. He raised an eyebrow and cracked a wry smile. "Too close," he said, shaking his head. "Too close."

Despite the lightheartedness of the blowgun contest, I could see the strain and fatigue of struggle on the faces of the meeting participants. These people wanted desperately to prevent the destruction of tribal culture in Brazil and to retain some decent tribal lands. But every day they lost ground, lost land, and lost lives. They knew the clock was ticking on their heritage.

THE
SHAMAN'S
CURE

If Manaus is the gateway to the Brazilian Amazon, Antonio Matas is a gatekeeper. Back in Manaus from Boa Vista, Bernie and I visited Antonio at his large, prominent shop at the bustling Mercado Antonio Lisboa, whose marble floors were worn down by a century of footprints. Antonio is the local curandero, a sought-after advisor who dispenses plant medicines. Medicine collectors deliver a variety of medicinal barks, leaves, and roots to Antonio's shop, where he can be found recommending botanicals for a sluggish liver, high blood pressure, or poor libido. "This is a very convenient place," Antonio said to Bernie and me. "You don't have to go off into the bush. There are many good medicines here." He is equally at ease with patients or the TV crews from all over the world that flock to his shop to shoot news segments and documentaries about medicinal plants from the world's greatest forest. On our first visit to see Antonio, a Japanese crew was filming his array of medicinal plants.

Catuaba and Muirapuama, American-Style

In the United States, you'll most commonly find catuaba and muira-puama in capsule form. Capsules are convenient and effective. I, however, always prefer to take herbs in their more traditional form when it's not oner-ously difficult to do so. Therefore, I recommend getting catuaba and muira-puama in the "loose herb" form, in this case the powdered barks. (You'll find sources for doing this in Resources on page 281.) Catuaba and muirapuama are woody tasting and present no offensive flavor barrier.

I asked Antonio Matas, the most respected herbalist in Manaus, what the best way is to take catuaba and muirapuama. He recommended simply mixing a teaspoon of the combined powdered barks in about three fingers of water and drinking it once daily. "You will have the sexual vitality of a much younger person," he told me.

To make the mixture even more potent, you can add a teaspoon of pow-dered guarana (*Paullinia cupana*).

Another option: Some people in the Amazon rain forest soak a handful of the barks of catuaba and muirapuama for 3 weeks in wine, and then strain and drink the resulting herbal infusion. "You can drink a glass of that wine every day," Antonio says. "It will make you sexually very strong."

I needed to devote much of the rest of my stay in the Amazon to learning more about the two widely employed sex-enhancers catuaba and muirapuama. Medicine-hunting means not only knowing all you can about the properties and uses of a plant, but also understanding the extent of its availability and the chain of its trade from the jungle to market. By starting with Antonio—the market—we were actually working backward.

The timing of our trip to the Amazon to investigate catuaba and muirapuama was in part dictated by the Viagra craze. Though clearly effective, Viagra's side effects exact too stiff a penalty for achieving a good erection. As a result, demand is rising for safe, natural aphrodisiacs that would be valuable not just for men but for women as well. "There is nothing that compares with catuaba and muirapuama together," Antonio said, echoing what the shaman Nazareth had told me on our first trip up the river. "I have used these plants with hundreds of people. The old become sexually young again. Impotent men can have sex for the first time in years. Even healthy couples find that these plants put extra fire in their sex lives." Women too? I asked. "Yes, definitely for women too," he answered. "Many women—not just men—come in here for increased sexual energy. Catuaba and muirapuama help them both." Then I asked Antonio if he used the two himself. He smiled. "Sometimes."

Even before Nazareth and Antonio Matas (among others) had confirmed it, we had learned that few reputed health-enhancing plants are as popular or as widely consumed among the natives of the northern Amazon River basin as the barks of the catuaba tree (*Erthyroxylum catuaba*) and the muirapuama tree (*Ptychopetalum olacoides*). Both have been widely used by natives and non-natives for centuries to increase libido and improve sexual potency. The common use of catuaba and muirapuama as a blend illustrates the centuries-old native skill in combining plants to achieve specific health effects.

The harvesting and sale of these two plants is big business throughout Brazil, so I asked Antonio how the supply was holding up in the forest area near Manaus. He shook his head. "Actually, that's a problem," he said. "There used to be lots of those trees around, but the medicines have become so popular that many have been cut down. You can still find the trees, but it's not like it used to be." Bernie asked if anybody was cultivating the two trees. "Yes, in Rondonia," Antonio replied, referring to another Amazon region state farther south. "That's the only way we're going to prevent them from completely disappearing. More and more people want better sexual health, so there is going to be only increased demand."

Antonio was addressing a problem that is of increasingly greater concern as herbs become more popular. How do you obtain an adequate supply of valuable botanicals for a growing market without harvesting them to extinction? The answer, as Antonio said, lies in cultivation. For example, there used to be enough wild echinacea in North America to provide biomass for herbal remedies, but the great increase in that herb's popularity has made it necessary for growers to cultivate echinacea for herbal companies. The same is true with ginseng. Today, the vast majority of ginseng sold in the world is farmed. Goldenseal, another popular herb, has been so heavily picked in the wild that it's seriously endangered. Even in the immense Amazon, a preponderance of certain types of plants does not mean that they can be endlessly picked in the wild. They must be replenished. If medicinally valuable trees like catuaba and muirapuama are going to be popular sex-enhancing herbs into the future, they need to be produced in a sustainable manner.

Antonio's shop was filled with bags of dried herbs, neatly sealed packages of powdered guarana, catuaba, and muirapuama, and bottles containing elixirs for everything from fortifying nerves to improving digestion. There was also a line of labeled bins that contained neat pieces of cut and dried bark. One bin was full of murure (*Brosimum acutifolium*), used to relieve arthritis pain. Another bin contained carapanauba (*Aspidosperma excelsium*), which we'd seen in the wild upriver with Bernie's family. The catuaba and muirapuama bins were almost empty. "These two go the fastest of all," Antonio remarked.

Before heading back up the river, Bernie and I stayed at the Best Western Hotel in Manaus for 2 nights, which gave us an opportunity to check out the use of another popular Amazonian plant. We had seen dozens of guarana products at Antonio's shop, and guarana sodas were everywhere in Manaus. We found dozens of guarana stands serving mixed fruit smoothies with herbs. Brazil may be a huge coffee-producing nation, but guarana is the most adored caffeine-bearing plant of the country. Natives make a dried paste from the seeds of the bushy tree (*Paullinia cupana*), which grows both wild and cultivated in the upper Amazon basin. Guarana seed paste contains from 2.5 percent to 5 percent caffeine (coffee has 1 to 2 percent), and it's used in soft drinks, syrups, and guarana sticks. The sticks, which look like brown dynamite, are scraped on a grater, and the powder is put into beverages. At guarana stands, powdered guarana seed paste is added to blends of exotic fruits like acai, cupuacu, buriti, mango, and papaya, resulting in sweet, energizing fruit smoothies.

It's not just the natural lift that brings customers to the guarana stands, though. Every stand offers an herbal "super sex drink," which contains about a heaping teaspoon of powdered catuaba and muirapuama barks combined with another tea-

An Amazon Super Sex Drink

A great way to get the energy-boosting and sex-enhancing benefits of catuaba and muirapuama is to combine them with stimulating guarana, the caffeine-bearing, great-tasting seed from the northern Amazon. Just combine the following in a blender, mix until it's smooth, pour, drink, and enjoy.

1 cup of apple juice

1 banana

2 tablespoons of yogurt

1 teaspoon of catuaba bark powder

1 teaspoon of muirapuama bark powder

1 teaspoon of guarana seed powder

A dash of vanilla extract

spoon of guarana. At guarana stands, couples buy sex drinks together and smile at each other suggestively as they drink. Other men and women individually consume the herbal elixirs on the spot—and take more home in plastic bottles to their partners. The people who work at the stands have countless anecdotes to share. My favorite was about the 100-year-old man who consumed a sex drink and then went home and chased his equally aged wife around the bedroom. Though surely apocryphal, the story spoke to the place that these herbs hold in popular Brazilian culture.

I asked a young man behind the counter of one guarana bar if the herbal sex drinks really worked. "Oh, man," he replied. "You better have a date. These drinks make the sexual feelings very strong, and you can just go and go all night long." He took down jars of powdered guarana, catuaba, and muirapuama from a shelf and scooped a little of each onto a plate for us to taste. "We get so many people, especially couples, who come back here all the time for the sex drink," a young woman making blender drinks behind the bar piped in. "They wouldn't keep coming back if the drinks didn't work for them." A woman waiting for blender drinks at the counter remarked that the barks in the sex drinks were very special gifts from the rain forest, that a lot of trees were being cut down, and that a lot of native people were getting pushed out of their ancestral homes. "The forest must be protected, and the native people must be helped," she said. "Be sure to tell that to the people back in the United States."

THE VISION BLOSSOM

Bernie and I were ready to go back up the river to his family, where we planned to hike into the forest with Geronimo to see more catuaba and muirapuama as well as other medicinal plants he knows. Behind the market we found the boatman Pedro Roque, and this time he took us up the river without incident. Even though we had been away for only 8 days, we were greeted with big hugs and smiles by Bernie's relatives. We sat around and talked about Gilberto, Domingo, and the other Indians we met. Bernie told the caxiri story, and there was unanimous consent that we did the right thing by refraining from drinking Francisca's brew.

Bernie and I set off with María and José and their son Arnaud to visit a shaman named Raymunda, who lived in the forest several miles away. Our long boat with its small outboard motor made its way through a chaotic series of tiny waterways past large islands of grass that shifted the landscape as they came and disappeared. After about an hour, we stopped and climbed a hill, where an older woman was waiting to let us know that the shaman Raymunda had been called away. How, I wondered, did she or Raymunda know we were coming? With no phones, no mail, no couriers, no faxes, no e-mail—none of that—we'd had no way to announce our visit. Still, Raymunda had left this woman to greet us and express her regrets for having missed us.

According to the woman on the hill, a local Ipixuna woman had been sleeping around with a number of men, and then had made the near-fatal blunder of visiting a sacred area in her psychically impure state. Wrathful spirits caused her body to contort and her hands to gnarl. The victim was in agony, and Raymunda had been summoned at once to take care of the spirit-tormented woman. A shaman's work is never done. We would have to come back another time.

That afternoon, Bernie and I set off down the river with Arnaud and his brother Zezinho to collect lavender-colored muru blossoms. The native people of the Amazon use certain sacred or visionary plants for ritual purposes, for healing, to divine the future, to consecrate certain events, and to know the spirits that govern their world. According to José and Bernie, muru, the "vision blossom," is an important sacred plant for the Ipixuna. Muru is found in thick clusters of hardy green grass along the banks of the river. Supposedly, large muru blossoms have little potency; only the small, fresh blossoms are used.

The four of us trolled the edge of thick, floating grasses in a small wooden boat. We looked for clusters of wide, heart-shaped leaves. Within those clusters we found the small lavender muru blossoms. It was hot, buggy work, and we had to watch out for poisonous water snakes. We saw large, boat-tipping alligators slip beneath the water's surface as we edged along the grasses.

Muru is used by the Ipixuna people around mid-September—the beginning of spring—to worship the land and to petition the great spirit for a bountiful harvest. After land has been prepared for planting, a family elder lights a small pile of dried muru blossoms. Carrying the smoking flowers, he walks over the area to be planted, spreading the smoke much in the same manner that incense is used to infuse a church with its aromatic vapors. The ashes of the burnt blossoms are scattered on a portion of ground, after which women bring crop seeds for planting. They chant prayers to Caapora, the god of flora, and make offerings of fruit and seeds. The elder then drinks a potion made from the freshly squeezed leaves of young muru blossoms. In about 45 minutes, a feeling of happiness starts to come over him as the psychoactive effects of the plant kick in. Sometimes, the elder will also smoke dried blossoms of muru. Through this ceremony, the elder is granted a blessing from the spirits, which is auspicious for the health of the crops that will be planted. It is through this kind of ritual use of mind-altering plants that native people gain direct access to the spirit world.

I wonder, however, about the claims of psychoactivity for this particular plant. Known widely as water hyacinth (*Eichornia crassipes*), muru is a common ornamental plant worldwide. There is no information describing any psychoactivity to be found in the scientific literature. Unfortunately, the samples I collected molded, so I didn't have the opportunity to experiment with the plant myself. If the young blossoms of common water hyacinth are psychoactive, why hasn't this been previously noted? If not, what accounts for the Ipixunas' use of the plant to induce happiness and elicit a blessing from the spirits? Whatever it is, this isn't the first case of science and indigenous experience being at odds.

A CATUABA HUNT

"You know, I don't smell any fresh coffee," Bernie said, back in the shack around 5:00 in the afternoon. "I think I'll go tell María that you want her to make you a fresh pot. She's already talking about what kind of fish she's going to make for you for dinner. I might as well take advantage of that." As Bernie headed off to proposition María for coffee in my name, I called out, "You're a mean man, Bernie." He looked back and grinned. "I know." A moment later, Bernie came back into the room, with María pointing at him. "I got found out," Bernie hung his head. "And you know, it's all your fault, big guy." María came to my defense, telling Bernie, "Chris wouldn't ask me to make him food, even if he was starving." Then she went off to make that fresh pot of coffee. "You know, brother," Bernie shared thoughtfully, "I used to lie around pretending to have a fever, just so María would make coffee. After a while, the trick didn't work."

The next morning, Bernie and I climbed into the motorboat with José and his son Theley and headed across the river to Geronimo's shack. We arrived at a dilapidated, crumbling structure with a partially caved-in roof, leaning walls, and a tilting, rotted porch. The river was up to the floorboards. Geronimo stood on the porch, shirtless and smiling, surrounded by dogs, cats, chickens, and a monkey. Geronimo's wife, Lady D., came to the door in an incongruous slinky red dress. "You see, brother," Bernie told me, "the indigenous people on this river, they are very poor. But also some of them are just strange." We pulled alongside the shack and stepped onto the porch, gingerly avoiding holes, split boards, and animal crap. "You need a new house, man," Bernie told Geronimo. "Yeah," Geronimo acknowledged. "Maybe in less than one season, this whole shack will fall down. Then we'll have no place to live. But I don't have the money for a new one. I have cut down some trees for lumber, but I can't afford to get a house built."

José explained to Geronimo that we wanted to go out into the forest to see catuaba and muirapuama. Geronimo pulled on some rubber boots and a short-sleeved shirt open in the front, and he was ready. We boated from Geronimo's shack to some elevated ground nearby and tied the boat to a tree. From there we walked single file along a narrow path that went from an open, grassy area into the darkness of the forest. As we walked, cicada buzzed, birds called, lizards scampered. José turned to me. "Be very careful of snakes," he said. "Only walk where I walk." In single file with Geronimo in the lead, we followed the path until it ceased to exist. Then we maneuvered through the forest, ducking low-hanging vines, giving broad berth to large nests of wasps, and watching out for thorns and hanging snakes. Blue morpho butterflies fluttered by gracefully, and mosquitoes swarmed us in hungry clouds.

"You know, man," Bernie said, "I got bitten one time by a green snake, right on the side of my neck. They like to go for this area. He was hanging from a tree, and he bit me. I got sick, but thank the great spirit I didn't die. I think it was a dry bite." Dry bites, not uncommon, occur when poisonous vipers sink their fangs into a person or animal, but inject no venom. A dry bite can convey septic bacteria that may cause an infection or illness, but it won't usually kill the recipient. Still, snakebites are the number one cause of accidental death in the Amazon rain forest. Woodsmen like Geronimo and José remain ever alert to the presence of snakes, and even to the smell of their scat.

The forest was relatively easy to navigate, since it lacked much underbrush. But it was dark due to the low, medium, and high canopies of various trees, which competed for and shaded out almost all sun. We skirted muddy and wet areas. "We are going to pay tribute to the mother catuaba tree," Geronimo told us as we hiked farther into the green woods, with its hanging lianas and monkey calls. Along the way we passed serungueira, or rubber trees (*Hevea brasiliensis*), with diagonal slash marks where tappers had cut the bark to collect latex for sale to rubber traders. We saw a number of tall rosewood trees (*Aniba rosaeodora*), which are cut for timber or are chipped and steam-distilled to yield linalol-rich rosewood oil, which is used in perfumery and toiletries and aromatherapy. "We're lucky to see these," Bernie remarked. "People cut them down everywhere." There was carapanauba, with its stomach-soothing medicinal bark. It is also commonly used for canoe paddles, and is therefore called paddle wood. At a giant kapoc tree, Theley thumped the great buttressed hollow trunk, which resonated like a huge ceremonial drum.

Bernie pointed out edible fruits, including Brazil nuts (*Bertholletia excelsa*), the red berries of wild guarana with their protruding black eyelike seeds, and the fruits of the acai palm, which hung from the trees like cascading strands of curtain beads. As we walked, Bernie spotted a couple of brown capuchin monkeys up in a tree and pointed out a nervous agouti, a cat-size rodent, bounding away from us. One of the forest's avian beauties, a vibrant red catinga, flew by. Numerous parrots squawked and soared overhead. "Look up there." José pointed to a tree limb, around which a fat boa was coiled. All around us lizards scampered up and down trees.

As we moved on, a stream of leaf-cutter ants, all carrying pieces of leaves on their backs, paraded across our path. Hundreds of different varieties of beetles, large and small, moved up and down trees or crawled on the forest floor. We saw several huge centipedes. "Watch out for those guys, man," Bernie warned. "If one of those bites you, you will get very sick." Tiny white orchids, pink and white striated orchids, and gold and green varieties punctuated the emerald forest with vibrant color. Spiny bromeliads gave a flamingo-hued shock to the woods. Scents of all kinds teased our olfactory senses, from floral to animal, fruity to fecal. All around, huge termite colonies thrived. Geronimo pointed out several vines, including *Banisteriopsis caapi*, which is mixed with any of a number of other plants, including the leaves of *Psychotria viridis*, to make a potent hallucinogenic drink called ayahuasca. The active hallucinogenic substance in the potion, N,N-dimethyltryptamine, produces powerful visions. Shamans and healers use ayahuasca to divine knowledge, to effect healings, and for vision quests. Another vine Geronimo showed us is used to make fish poison. The vine is boiled in water, which is then dumped into the river. The vine preparation suffocates the fish, which float to the surface of the water and are collected.

We came upon a small muirapuama tree, and Geronimo stopped to run his hand along the bark. "In this area, there are many of these," he said. "In other places, they have all been cut down." José explained that collectors would go through the forest felling muirapuama trees, floating them out on the river, and grinding them up in mills. Now, after a couple of miles of sweaty, mosquito-bitten hiking, we came to a magnificent, straight tree, which rose a good 100 feet from the forest floor. "The mother catuaba tree," José told us.

José and Geronimo walked around the tree, picking up leaves from the ground and placing them up against the trunk. All the while they repeated something in Ipixuna. Bernie and I also placed leaves. After a couple of minutes of this, we stopped, and Geronimo spoke in a solemn tone in Crinicoru. When he was finished, Bernie translated: "He has just asked the spirits to bless this tree and to keep it safe. Geronimo says that this tree is the mother of the catuaba trees in this area. He says that it is very important that this tree stays alive, and that nobody cuts it down. He also says that he and José know these woods very well, and if anybody tries to cut down this tree, they will protect it. This tree is sacred. If it goes, the spirits will be very upset."

Then Bernie flashed a crooked smile. "You know, brother," he said, "Geronimo just said all that in Crinicoru, not in Ipixuna, just to annoy José. But José is not going to say anything. Geronimo is just provoking him." I admired the great reach of the grand catuaba tree, with its leafy branches high in the sky, and hoped that it would remain standing tall and healthy. I shot several photographs of the tree, and of Bernie, José, Geronimo, and Theley.

José told us, "Now that we have come to the mother catuaba tree and have paid our respects to the spirits of the forest, we can go look at some other catuaba trees." We walked a little farther into the forest, and in a few places came upon straight, tall catuaba trees, though none as large as the mother tree. Later in the day, we headed back toward the river, stopping to look at more trees and wildlife, passing numerous catuaba and muira-puama, and spotting sloths and howler monkeys.

Back at Geronimo's shack, we thanked him for his help. He scratched his shirtless belly and said that he liked being in the forest. I looked at the sad condition of his home and imagined that it couldn't cost too much to help him get a new one built. I broached this idea to Bernie. "Oh yeah, man, I bet you could do that real cheap," he agreed. "But for Geronimo, whatever that would cost, even if it is just a small amount of money, would be completely impossible." When I told Geronimo that I would be happy to help him, he said he knew a man who would build a new shack for him—a really good one—if he had a little money. We all decided that the best thing was for Geronimo to bring that man around to José and María's shack, where we could work something out.

That evening around 8:30, Geronimo came paddling over to the shack in a small, leaky canoe, shirtless and grinning in the mosquito dark. With him was a slender, wiry woodcutter and carpenter named Domingo. "That was fast," Bernie told Geronimo. "Yeah, well, my house is falling down," he said. "And if Chris can help me, then I want to talk about it." The four of us shook hands and sat down, surrounded by José and María and all the rest of the family in the closed shack. Bernie, reclining in his hammock and presiding over the meeting with Geronimo and Domingo by candlelight, reminded me of Marlon Brando in *The Godfather*.

Geronimo's shack, it was agreed, was soon going to fall into the river. "You're going to be swimming with the alligators," is how Bernie put it. "I don't think Lady D. is going to like that too much." Domingo said he was a capable carpenter who could build a good, strong house for Geronimo. José and Geronimo knew of work that Domingo had done, and they confirmed that he was the man for the job. Bernie asked Domingo how much money it would cost to cut the wood and build a solid house for Geronimo, Lady D., and all their animals. Domingo stared at the floor a while. After much consideration, he said he could do the whole job for 100 *reales*. Sixty dollars.

Since Geronimo didn't know denominations of money, Bernie suggested that José act as the treasurer of Geronimo's home-building project, with $20 paid to Domingo in advance to get started. José said, "I'll do that for Geronimo, even though he's a Crinicoru." Bernie turned to me. "You hear that, big guy?" he asked. "This goes back and forth between these men for a whole lifetime. They will never leave it alone." Domingo was happy for the job and promised to build a good house. Geronimo was so grateful he could hardly speak. "When that house is built," he told me, "every time I walk inside I will think of you."

I found out months later that Domingo had done a fine job, and that Geronimo's new house was so sturdy and well-built that Lady D.'s family had moved in. Geronimo still spent many nights sleeping in the forest, tied to a tree limb in the upper canopy.

RAYMUNDA'S CURE

Late one afternoon, a man in a small motorboat arrived at the shack. I hadn't seen him before. He stepped out of his boat and onto the porch, and spoke with José. After a few minutes he tipped his straw hat, got back into his boat, and motored off. José came inside, where Bernie was resting in his hammock and I was writing in my trip journal. "That man says that shaman Raymunda wants to see you tomorrow," he told me. Raymunda, he had said, would be found in a different place than where we had previously sought her out.

The next morning, José, Theley, Bernie, and I hopped into the long boat with the outboard and headed off to see Raymunda. This time we took a different route. We traveled an hour up the nearby Paracuruba River, and then cut into a small channel and headed for a couple of miles into thick jungle. At one point we stopped at a shack and asked an old woman who was vigorously cleaning fish with a knife where Raymunda could be found. A couple more miles into the woods, she replied, pointing up the small waterway, or igarape. Eventually the waterway became narrow and clogged with floating vegetation, forcing us to stop repeatedly to untangle the propeller. Hawks large and small sat atop trees, soared over hills, glided into marshes, and winged past our boat. There must have been plenty of small creatures to eat in the area.

Several times it seemed we had boated our way to a dead end, but there was always a narrow waterway affording just enough room to squeeze through. A few times we pulled at tall grass on both sides of the boat to move ourselves forward. In slightly wider spots we motored along carefully at a slow pace, winding around giant trees and thick stands of tall, broad-leafed marsh plants. After half an hour more of slow, difficult maneuvering, we came to a steep hill with a stairway hewn out of a red clay hillside. At the top of the hill stood a shack, where we could see an old woman, a man and woman in their thirties, a young boy and girl, several cute, mangy puppies, and a few chickens.

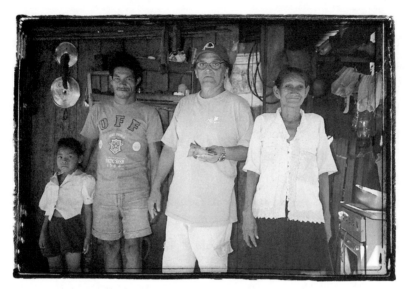

Shaman Raymunda (right), Ipupiara, and cured carpenter and his child

The old woman turned out to be the shaman Raymunda, who said she was glad we got her message and that she was sorry she had missed us when we came to see her before. She explained that she was staying at this particular shack for a few days, performing healing work for nearby people. The man with her, a carpenter from Manaus, was a Raymunda healing success story. He had been suffering from back problems that became so debilitating he was eventually unable to work and feed his family. He had been examined and treated by a doctor in Manaus, but he only got worse. As a last resort he sought out Raymunda, traveling with his wife and two children to see her. She treated him intensively with teas, baths, poultices, and rituals for a few days, and his back was so improved that he intended to head back to Manaus and to work. "When I came here, I could barely stand," he told us. "Now my back feels good and strong again. Raymunda has saved me and my family."

A small, thin woman with weathered cocoa skin and an attentive, kind manner, Raymunda invited us to sit in her shack and have some coffee. Laundry hung along one wall, pans and utensils on another. A row of tin cups rested on a wooden shelf, and a broom hung from a rafter. Bernie made the usual introductions, telling Raymunda who we were, where we came from, and that we were interested in the skills and knowledge of shamans. We had heard that she was very talented, and so that's why we had sought her out. Raymunda listened as though she already knew all of this, but she allowed Bernie the formality of saying it. She told us that, yes, many people came to see her. The spirits had blessed her with abilities, and she had also been taught a lot about medicinal plants from several great teachers. "I also perform many rituals to the spirits, to honor them, and to protect the people and the forest," she said.

After this introductory conversation, Raymunda asked me to sit on a small wooden bench. "I am going to get in touch directly with your spirit," she said. "There is something you need, not just information." With that she began to chant softly in Ipixuna, while touching me just as Edna had, but without a plant in her hand. Her diagnosis and prescription were much the same as Edna's as well—envious people were interfering with my business at home and I was to take evening baths with the plants mané velho and cheirro cheiroso.

Raymunda turned her attention to Bernie, instructing him to sit on the wooden bench. She went through the same process of chanting softly while touching Bernie lightly on his head, face, shoulders, chest, and neck. When she was finished, she looked at him with sadness in her eyes. "You have suffered a lot over the past several years." Bernie hung his head and began to cry softly.

"It has been unbelievably hard for me," he offered. "And for my wife, too. It is such a struggle." Raymunda put a hand on Bernie's shoulder. "You are almost through this very difficult time. The most important thing is to have faith in the spirits and re-member what you were taught. You can regain the power you have lost, but you must walk back to the spirits. You must come back from where you have gone."

Many of the medicinal plants Raymunda used were ones we'd learned about either from Nazareth or Geronimo. She told us that she got particularly good relief for arthritis pain with murure bark, which we had seen at Antonio's place in Manaus. Helecho (*Lycopodium cernuum*) could be used in a bath to ward off negative spirits as well as to relieve arthritis pain. I asked her about catuaba and muirapuama, and received the familiar an-swer. "Those are the very best for sex," she said. "Many impotent men recover and become sexually active, and people who have lost all sexual interest feel young again. If you use catuaba and muirapuama, you become sexually strong." She confirmed that soaking the barks in a glass of water was an efficacious method for taking the plants.

When it was time for us to leave, I offered Raymunda some money, so she could afford to heal people without concern for how she would take care of herself. She was reluctant, but I ex-plained that I wasn't paying her for her help. She smiled and took the money, and gave me a pat on the shoulder. "Go with the blessings of the spirits," she said. "You are always welcome here, and I will ask the spirits to watch over both of you."

THE ELDEST SHAMAN

The next day, Geronimo showed up at the shack just in time for morning coffee, with a sack of cut, dried bark in his canoe. "Catuaba," he told us. Geronimo sat shirtless in his canoe, drinking a cup of coffee and smoking a hand-rolled cigarette. He explained that he had cut the catuaba bark from some trees and dried it in the sun, and that a buyer from near Manaus would come around in a boat any day now and pay him for the bark after weighing it. "This is part of how these people make a living," Bernie commented. "Just like José will sell some fish for a little money, and they all sell the vegetables and manioc and melons they grow during the dry season. Some, like Geronimo, also collect different medicinal plants that are popular in the markets, and every so often a buyer will show up in a boat and buy the plants."

Later on, María asked Bernie, "Does Chris know about María Sena?" Bernie said he didn't think so and asked me, "Do you know about that shaman who is more than 100 years old?" I asked Bernie just how he thought I would know about her—a news brief on The Shaman Channel? "Hey, man, I don't know," he came back. "I just thought maybe you came across her in conversation somehow. In any case, she is the most respected and oldest shaman around here. José's sister Paula saw her recently, and she invited us to go to see her. Paula says that María Sena is 103 years old, but that she is more powerful than any of the other shamans around here." I told Bernie that I was keen to visit her. "Maybe we'll go tomorrow," he replied.

The next morning after coffee and pan-fried bread, José, Bernie, Paula, Theley, and I climbed into the motorboat and set off upriver. We traveled for an hour or so, passing riverboats, canoes, and children bathing. Women sat on floating planks, beating laundry and cleaning fish. Black and pink dolphins breached ahead of us, vultures soared huge overhead, and alligators floated by tall grass, patiently waiting for food to come by. Fish splashed on the surface of the water as we cruised along, the wind in our hair.

At one point, we cut into a small igarape and motored deep into the forest. Soon we emerged into a large, secluded lagoon, riotously alive with hawks, herons, luminous blue birds that flitted from bush to bush, orange and black butterflies, blue morphos, splashing fish, and spectacular flowers. We traveled the full length of the recondite lagoon and into the woods again, cruising slowly and carefully through another narrow, heavily forested waterway, and emerging eventually into a small river. We moved along the river for a while, and then stopped at a small mooring by a hill. Paula climbed out and walked up the hill to a shack. A few minutes later, she returned to the boat and made a waving gesture downriver. "We have to go farther that way," she announced. This was the beginning of the game called Find María Sena.

We continued down the narrow river to another shack. Paula got out, spoke with a woman who was cleaning fish on some planks, and announced, "María Sena was here, but now she has gone to another place." We eventually came to a patch of elevated land where a man who looked like Emiliano Zapata's double labored in the sun. He held a machete in one hand, and sweat soaked his grimy T-shirt. We got out of the boat and shook hands with him. From inside a small shack, a woman emerged— María Sena's daughter Martha, who at 72 was her mother's youngest child. "Oh, I'm so sorry my mother is not here," she said. "She has gone to lead a gathering of shamans deep in the forest. If you wish, you can come back on Monday, and she will be here." Before we left, Martha showed us a small, humble chapel María Sena used for healings. On an altar-table sat a hand-carved white dove. It occurred to me that even though both men and women are shamans in the Amazon, Bernie and I had encountered only women shamans. There was no particular reason for that as far as we could tell. It's just the way things worked out.

On Monday, Bernie, José, Theley, Paula, and I made the same long, picturesque trip to María Sena's. Emiliano Zapata was still laboring in the broiling sun, but he stopped and gave us a big smile and pointed his machete toward the little chapel. Martha emerged from the house to greet us, and she walked us over to the chapel, where we found a tiny, mocha-colored old woman with long, thick gray hair. María Sena, barefoot in a green floral print dress, extended small smooth hands and took ours in them one by one. Her wrinkled face was marvelously expressive, and when she made eye contact, she seemed to be gazing directly at my soul. She invited us to sit down and get comfortable.

"I was at a gathering of shamans when you came the other day," she told us. "I knew you would come today, so I

103-year-old shaman María Sena and her daughter Martha

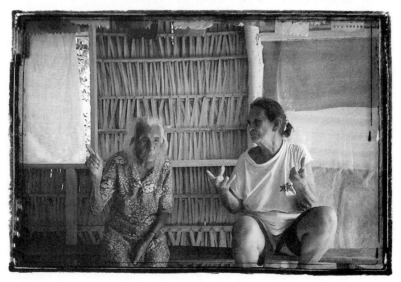

made sure to be here." Paula said it was no trouble to come back, and that we were happy to be able to see her. The old shaman nodded. "We have gatherings once in a while, where all the shamans get together to heal the forest and to help protect people," she said. "We stay together for a few days, and we perform ceremonies and healings. Most of the shamans have no students. The younger people do not want to learn this traditional knowledge. When the shamans die, the old knowledge will disappear."

María Sena knew about Bernie from when he had lived with the Ipixuna before moving to the United States. "This is my first time back in 10 years," he told her. "That is too long," she said. "You must come back to the river and the forest and the spirits. You must come back here to breathe the air and drink the water and see your people." Bernie told María Sena that he understood, but that he had been unable to get back to the Amazon for lack of funds. "If you will use your power, you can come back as much as you wish," she replied.

We talked for a while longer, and then Bernie asked if María Sena would diagnose me and perform any healing that was necessary. María Sena readily agreed. As I sat in a chair, she approached me, uttered a few words in Ipixuna, and placed her hands on my head. I was surprised by the strength of her hands. The sensation I got was that of being touched firmly by someone a quarter her age. She moved her hands about my head—side to side, front and back, front and top—pressing both palms on me. She laid her firm hands on my shoulders, pressed a palm against the center of my chest, and put her hands back on my head, all the while softly chanting.

When María Sena's hands were on my head, I felt a vibration and assumed that her hands were trembling. But when I looked, they didn't appear to be shaking even slightly. I felt a sensation in my head, as though the insides of my skull bones were warming up. She finished the session by pulling firmly on my fingers, and for the third time I was told I had the evil eye on me. And for the third time, I was prescribed baths with mané velho and cheirro cheiroso. "But above all else," María Sena said, "you must remember the spirits and honor them. Then you can easily go from one world to another." I asked her what she meant. "You go from your world to this one, and then back again," she answered. "This is your work. You are a bridge. For this reason, you must remember the spirits always."

Now Bernie sat in the same spot where I had sat, and she performed a similar routine of chanting, touching, and pressing him with her palms. When she was finished, she told Bernie that he had lost a lot of power, and that circumstances in his life had drained him of energy and hope. "You are right," Bernie confided. "I feel all beaten up, just trying to make ends meet in Washington. It's very hard." María Sena told Bernie that things would start to change. "The worst times are almost over," she assured him. "You will have better days soon. You will come back to the spirits. But you must never stay away for long again. You need to come here, so you will always remember, and you will always be close to the spirits."

As I watched and listened to María Sena, the inside of my skull was getting hot, like an electric stove coil turned to high. María Sena looked at me for a moment and decided to perform more work. As I sat, she made similar motions as before, chanting all the while. The heat in my head subsided, and I felt curiously detached, as though some perceptual shift had just taken place. "You will feel many things," María Sena told Bernie and me. "Tonight I will perform a healing ritual at midnight for both of you. This is an especially powerful night, so the effect of the ritual will be very strong."

After more conversation, warm goodbyes, and an invitation from María Sena to come back any time, we got back into the motorboat. I waved goodbye to Zapata, who smiled and waved his machete. As we set off for home, my head cooked with internal heat, and I felt only half inside my body. "Do you feel completely strange?" I asked Bernie. "You know what I feel like?" he replied. "I feel like one of those hot air balloons, with hot gas in it to make it go higher and higher, up in the very thin atmosphere." I knew exactly what he meant. "Do you think you've lost power?" I asked Bernie. "Yeah, I've known that for quite a while," he said. "I needed that teaching that María Sena gave. I must never stay away so long. It is heartbreaking. And then after a while, I don't even realize what I have forgotten."

By the time we got back to the shack later that afternoon, Bernie and I both felt on fire from the waist up. We immersed ourselves in the river, which cooled us down only briefly. Mostly, though, we cooked. María made buriti, the rich, creamy orange drink from the fruits of the *Mauritia flexuosa* palm. The buriti was sweet and delicious, but I felt as though I were drinking it in an oven. We lay around in our hammocks, and I had the sensation of roasting on a spit. Into the evening and the night, Bernie and I cooked and sweated, periodically checking in with each other. Long past when the windows were closed against the mosquito dark, I lay awake sweating in my hammock. In the middle of the night, exhausted from unabated inner heat, I succumbed to a deep sleep. In my dreams I was immersed in the river, drifting past creatures large and small and melting into the liquid current.

The next day, Bernie and I shared our experiences. "You know, brother, I felt like I was a roasting pig," Bernie shook his head. "But then very late I got so tired from the heat, I fell asleep. And do you know that I dreamed about the spirits? There was a great jaguar spirit. It came right up to me in the forest. And then in the river there was a dolphin spirit. And when I called out 'Ipupiara! Ipupiara!' the dolphins came to me, and they jumped all around."

Both of us felt right as rain, rested and somehow more solid. We agreed that María Sena had done something powerful. "This kind of thing," Bernie said, "can go on and on in your life, having a positive effect. I think that old lady did something very precious for us."

The day before Bernie and I were to leave the river, we wrapped plant samples, got our equipment together, and packed our freshly cleaned laundry—with cracked and smashed buttons, courtesy of the indomitable Nonata. In the afternoon, José took us over to Geronimo's dilapidated shack. Cats, dogs, and a pig wandered around on the cramped, broken porch. Lizards clung to the shack walls. Geronimo, half out of the doorway, snatched his young pet monkey by the tail and stepped out to greet us. The monkey screamed, grabbed onto Geronimo's fingers, and bit down hard, with no apparent effect. Geronimo just held its tail and stroked its head, and the monkey settled down. We told Geronimo that we would be leaving the next day, and we wanted to say goodbye.

We talked for about half an hour, and I thanked Geronimo for all of his help and friendship. He thanked me for helping him to build a new house. "When it is finished, you can come stay any time you want," he said. "You are always welcome in my home." After taking a few photographs, we shook hands with Geronimo and got back into José's boat. As we pulled away, Geronimo stood waving goodbye from his rotting porch, surrounded by animals, the grin of a wild man on his face, contentedly at one with the spirits of the river.

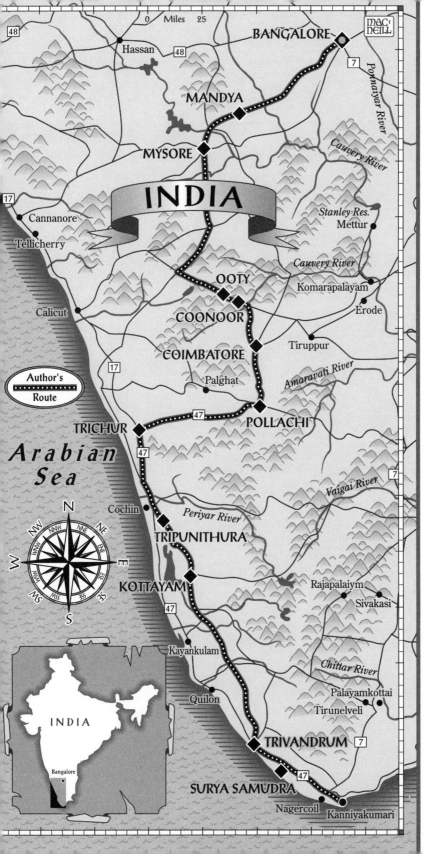

Medicine of the Gods

THE FOUR-LIMBED GOD

Afte a cramped and tiring 28 hours of flying and layovers
from Boston to Zurich to Bombay to Bangalore, we walked
down the gangway of an Indian Airways jet into an unseasonably
cool May morning for south India—only 80°F. Beyond shimmering jet fuel vapors fuming up from the tarmac, tall coconut
palms swayed, their lustrous green fronds dancing in a light
breeze.

Bangalore is a high-tech center, India's Silicon Valley. We
intended, however, to explore not silicon chips but an ancient
tradition. This city of roadside Siva temples and carts pulled by
oxen with jingling bells on their horns—as well as offices of
major computer corporations—would be our starting point on
another leg of the medicine trail. My wife Shahannah and I
would wend our way in a southerly direction investigating
Ayurveda, India's ancient system of natural medicine, which is a
fertile repository of medicinal herb uses that most Americans are
only beginning to recognize. We planned to visit growers of
medicinal plants, manufacturers of Ayurvedic herbal remedies,
and clinics where the methods of Ayurveda are practiced. As

such journeys go, it would be a reasonably comfortable one, requiring no stays in the jungle, no long periods away from basic amenities.

Our trip to south India was timely. In the 1960s and 1970s, some members of India's scientific community and the popular media expressed the notion that Ayurvedic medicines—India's traditional plant-based remedies—were passé. Herbs, they argued, should be replaced by technologically developed drugs. Ayurveda's patron god Dhanwantari should forfeit his heavenly post and be supplanted by a new god named science. Modernists argued that taking this great leap forward would help India shrug off its archaic image.

Even as this sector of India's intelligencia was making funeral arrangements, however, the god of science blessed the efficacy of Ayurvedic medicines. The same marvelous analytical tools and methods used to develop new drugs were plumbing the complex chemical secrets of purportedly beneficial plants and assessing their biological activity. Thin-layer chromatography enabled botanists to establish "fingerprint" identifications of medicinal plants. High-pressure liquid chromatography and mass spectrometry enabled them to examine chemical profiles of plants, identify specific substances, and determine their concentrations. Previously unavailable physiological testing methods helped investigators to evaluate the biochemical activities of plants and compounds from them.

The resulting flood of scientific studies and books revealed that Ayurvedic remedies work extraordinarily well, and that traditional formulas devised thousands of years ago do exactly what they are supposed to do. The god of science bowed at the altar of Dhanwantari, and remedies from the plant kingdom retained their noble position. Today, plant-based Ayurvedic remedies remain the primary medicines of India, with powerful support from both the government and the scientific community. The "science of life" is now the topic of major pharmacy conferences, and Ayurveda is a thriving, fashionable, much-discussed health phenomenon in the media. It's sexy. It's now. All the stars are into it.

At the airport we were met by H. Prakash, a guide who would assist us for the next 2 weeks, and a friendly looking driver. Prakash, a natty and fit-looking man in his early thirties, wore his hair short and cut a handsome figure with a well-trimmed moustache. We would come to discover that Prakash was a man of fastidious attention to detail—and an invaluable aid to our work.

Prasad, the driver, was only 21 and so slender that he appeared to have no hips. His thick black hair bordered a clipped full facial beard that climbed his face like moss. We would quickly discover that Prasad was a maniacal daredevil of a driver, who negotiated the road with a rare indifference toward danger or loss of life. With the aid of both men, we stowed our compact luggage in the back of a Tata Sumo, an Indian sport utility truck virtually identical in form, function, and discomfort to an early model Isuzu Trooper.

You can get away with stashing just a few items in an overnight bag if you're only going off to New York. But investigating natural medicine throughout south India for a few weeks requires diverse equipment, and we had packed with care and forethought. I won't say that we carried the world on our backs, but following the time-honored exhortations of the Boy Scouts, we were prepared.

Gadgets were high on our packing list for south India. My cameras and equipment included a Contax G1 autofocus with 28-millimeter, 45-millimeter, and 90-millimeter lenses and a flash; a small Contax TVS autofocus with a 28-millimeter to 56-millimeter zoom lens; 50 rolls of Kodak Ektachrome film; carrying and storage bags; air gun cleaners; cloths; more batteries than I needed; and a panoply of accoutrements. The Contax cameras, with their Zeiss lens, take crisp, brilliant shots. The auto-focus makes them close to idiot-proof, and the pictures they yield are marvelous. That helps when you have only precious seconds to fire off a shot of a moving elephant or a group of sari-clad women streaming down the street in a wave of brilliant silk. The photographs I would capture would be essential for presentation in the demanding schedule of seminars I conduct on natural medicines and the locations and cultures from which they originate.

I also packed a pocket-size Sony short-wave radio with tiny "turbo" headphones. The Sony runs on penlight batteries, and it's easy to noodle with late at night when the airwaves are crowded with Sri Lankan crooners, Burmese newscasts, Brazilian samba, BBC World News, Voice of Freedom broadcasts, Viennese symphonies, Christian missionaries, Bulgarian operas, Russian theater, and a thousand popular music programs from around the globe.

Shahannah was traveling with a Sony TRV900 digital video camera, 10 hours of digital video tape, power cords, international power converters, a recharger, carrying cases, and other miscellaneous electronic gear. With this video camera we would not only be able to capture exciting video, but we would have the option of taking brilliant digital still shots as well.

There was more than electronic equipment. I also carried a folding Gerber Gator knife and a larger Gerber tactical knife, luggage locks, Mini Mag flashlights, a compass, rope, maps, a journal, two travel books, pens, markers, labels, and a Leatherman multi-tool. For pure drinking water we carried a Katadyn filter, which offered insurance against contracting some perfectly ghastly water-borne diseases. After we carefully filtered water pure, we still treated it with iodine, just to make sure that any unwanted microbes that might somehow squeeze through a one-micron filtration barrier wound up dead and gone. Water purification alone does not spare a traveler from diseases in India, but it helps. You can still get plenty sick from food and insects, especially mosquitoes bearing either malaria or dengue.

This leads to our medical kit, which was chock-full of bandages, gauze, tape, syringes, unguents, ointments, antibacterial swabs, a simple surgical kit, and enough basic supplies to open a small but respectable bush clinic. We more often wound up using these supplies to help people we met, rather than for ourselves. We generally relied on herbs to meet our everyday health needs. As an anti-malarial, for example, we were taking capsules of the Chinese herb artemisia, which works every bit as well as pharmaceutical anti-malarials. But it's helpful to pack some high-caliber pharmaceutical ammo as well. We carried the broad spectrum antibiotic Ciprofloxacin in case of infection or a debilitating intestinal bacterial problem. We also were well-supplied with Imodium in the event of diarrhea, a condition so common in India that virtually every traveler there gets it sooner or later.

Add to all the goods described so far two well-stocked toiletry kits with all manner of dental care, shampoo, soaps, Q-tips, and so on, and clothing enough for 3 weeks on the road, covering varying terrain and climate. Much of our clothing was made by Ex Officio and was constructed of lightweight superfiber. Some came from august expedition outfitter Willis and Geiger. All of it was very good and took up little space. We were able to pack everything into one medium-size piece of Eagle Creek soft luggage each as well as one day pack each. We made sure to fly with all the irreplaceable electronic equipment in our carry-ons. Our footwear was sandals, which we wore on the plane. I carried a large wad of cash in a zippered wallet that looped on my belt and was hidden inside my pants. This precaution might at times have given the appearance of tumescence, but it did reduce the likelihood of theft.

In a gesture of considerable hospitality, Prakash invited us to the home of his in-laws for tea and breakfast before depositing us at our hotel. We sped off across town in the Tata Sumo with mad Prasad at the wheel. Trees and temples and tall buildings and tea stalls and tandoor parlors and tailor shops streamed by in vivid greens, reds, blues, yellows, and golds. Incense and diesel fumes and flowers and cow shit and cooking curries spilled a chaotic olfactory profusion. Temple bells rang, truck horns blared, high-voiced Hindu singers wailed loudly over tinny speakers, cow hooves clopped, scooter taxis sputtered, and India's fifth largest urban area roared into morning.

We stopped at a small apartment in a quiet, peaceful neighborhood of neat three-story buildings with colorful gardens and innumerable flowers and cacti on their porches. Inside we met Prakash's mother-in-law and father-in-law as well as his wife Vanita, with brilliant dark eyes and a serene manner that matched the gentle floating of her crimson silk sari cloth as she rustled about the apartment. Prakash and Vanita had lost their infant daughter to illness 2 years prior, and she was pregnant again and hopeful for the health of their next child. "Our daughter's death was very hard for us," Prakash said. "Especially for Vanita. She blamed herself, thinking that perhaps there was something she could have done. Then she blamed God for doing this thing to us. But these circumstances are not in our hands. It is God's decision who will live and who will die. Often we cannot understand why certain things in life occur. But everything is up to the will of God, not the will of man. By God's will only our next child will be strong and healthy. We pray for this."

As Prakash described his way of thinking and coping, he and Vanita sat close together on a small settee holding hands. Beside them a narrow teak-trimmed ceremonial table known as a puja closet was adorned with statues of Hindu gods, with offerings of rice, water, fresh marigold blossoms, and sticks of delicate champa incense, from which smoky tendrils curled through the air like lazy serpents. We ate rice and vegetables cooked with shredded coconut, and drank sweet tea.

After breakfast, we sped across town. In the lobby of our economical hotel, woozy versions of the Carpenters' greatest hits moaned from speakers in the ceiling. Karen Carpenter's voice rose and fell in an unsteady acoustic ellipse. It was apparently the only tape the hotel played, which they did around the clock. I wondered if employees bolted one by one in mad despair from this musical torture.

THE OLDEST MEDICINE

After a brief rest and a shower, Shahannah and I were picked up by Dr. S.K. Mitra, executive director of the Himalaya Drug Company, and Dr. Rangesh Paramesh, the company's medical advisor. While organizing our trip in the States, I had made contact with Dr. Mitra by e-mail, and he had promised to show us some of the key places of Ayurvedic practice in the Bangalore area. Himalaya Drug, India's largest provider of Ayurvedic remedies, founded in Dehra Dun in 1930, was the inspiration of M. Manal, who believed that the ancient system of Ayurveda could be brought into the modern world in a contemporary form through science and careful manufacturing processes.

As is so often the case, pure good fortune played a significant role in the early success of the fledgling company. On a trip to Burma, Manal observed that elephants were regularly fed a particular type of root, and he was told that the root had a calming effect on the large beasts. Intrigued, Manal brought samples of the plant back to India, where he conducted tests on its properties.

The plant, *Rauwolfia serpentina*, the source of the now widely used pharmaceutical alkaloid reserpine, demonstrated tranquilizing and anti-hypertensive properties. After a few years of rigorous testing, the product Serpina was launched. Serpina, the world's first-ever anti-hypertensive drug, was a great financial and health success, and it paved the way for further research and development of plant drugs. "Serpina was the very first product for Himalaya Drug," said Dr. Mitra. "Today we have more than 30 products, all very well researched and popular throughout all of India."

The day was broiling. Dr. Mitra and Dr. Paramesh wore dark, well-pressed business suits, crisp white shirts, and carefully knotted ties. Shahannah and I were in loose-fitting casual tropical clothing. Thus disparately attired, we headed off to our first destination in Bangalore, the Government Ayurvedic Medical College and its attached hospital, the Sri Jayachamarajendra Institute of Indian Medicine.

At the college, we were ushered into the office of Dr. S. M. Angadi, the director of Indian Systems of Medicine and Homeopathy. A group of curious staff members fluttered about, gesturing toward us with nods and speaking back and forth in Hindi. The spacious room, with a high ceiling, institutional green walls, gunmetal filing cabinets, a huge worn wooden desk, and several cushioned chairs, typified the offices of high-level Indian bureaucrats. It probably hadn't been remodeled since the Raj era of British colonial rule. Dr. Mitra introduced me and Shahannah as Mr. Chris and Mrs. Chris, names that would dog us like spaniels for the entire trip. At the same time, I realized I'd seldom get much more than a first-name initial to go with the last name of most people I met in India—even on their business cards—and often not even that.

After introductions and an offer of tea, Dr. Angadi invited us to sit and described the program at the college. "Our educational curriculum here is very specifically set up to guarantee the highest level of proficiency," he said. "Students must first complete 12 years of schooling, with all the basic sciences of biology, chemistry, and physics. They must do well in their studies, because it is a serious course to become an Ayurvedic physician. We offer a 5½-year program, with degrees in Ayurveda, Siddha, and Unani as well as a master's degree in yoga. Are you familiar with yoga?" I said that I practiced yoga daily and had done so for nearly 30 years, and this provoked exchanges of surprised glances and nods of approval in the office. "If you practice yoga," Dr. Angadi said with a warm smile, "then you understand how very important both the fitness of the body and the fitness of the spirit are to true health. If your body is infirm, and if your spirit is not in harmony, then there can be no true health. This is fundamental to our understanding."

I asked Dr. Angadi about the three systems of medicine he had mentioned. "Ah yes, you see, most people know only about Ayurveda, but there are the two others as well. Ayurveda developed out of the Aryan culture, which populated India long ago and whose original texts are in Sanskrit, the language of the Vedas. Siddha is the medicinal tradition of the Dravidians, who were the original inhabitants of the Indian subcontinent. All of the Siddha texts are written in Tamil, the ancient Dravidian language that is still widely spoken in south India today. Unani is the medicinal tradition brought here by the Mughul Empire. The Unani texts are written in classical Arabic, and the formulas still reflect the Arab culture and often feature sweet ingredients like raisins, honey, or sugar." Shahannah asked whether the three systems shared the same medicinal plants. "Oh, yes, yes," Dr. Angadi answered. "They have all adapted to the environment. Only plants that can be found here may be made into medicines. So today all three systems use the same medicinal plants. But the way the plants are prepared, and exactly what kinds of formulas are used, this will vary greatly."

From where I sat in Dr. Angadi's office, I could admire the craftsmanship of a colorful painting depicting a god with four arms. Accompanying the painting was a garland of fresh marigold blossoms. Dr. Angadi asked if I knew what I was looking at. I didn't. He invited Shahannah and me to the picture; Dr. Mitra and Dr. Paramesh followed. "This is the god Dhanwantari," he told us. "Dhanwantari is the presiding deity of Ayurveda. He watches over every aspect of this science of life, from the plants themselves to the doctors. This is why any time you go to a place where Ayurveda is practiced, whether they are making medicines or treating the sick, you will always find a picture or a statue of Dhanwantari. You will see this for yourselves as you travel around. The image of Dhanwantari reminds us always that only God gives the true gift of healing, and that we are just agents for that grace."

Dhanwantari, an aspect of the Hindu deity Vishnu, is always shown with four arms. One hand holds a leech for blood-letting, to facilitate recovery from disease. Another holds a small clay pot inside of which is a holy medicine, the precious elixir of longevity. A third hand holds a conch shell, which Dhanwantari uses to blow the cosmic Om, the sound of creation. By sounding this primordial tone, Dhanwantari creates awareness of holy truth in the world. In the fourth hand he holds a chacra, a spinning vortex of energy used to destroy darkness and ignorance, which are impediments to health and spiritual realization.

Hindus consider spiritual realization to be the true purpose of life in this world.

Ayurveda's origin in Vedic culture began around 5000 B.C., when concepts of surgery, herbalism, and diagnosis developed, along with an understanding of the principles of digestion, metabolism, and the specific nature of various diseases. The two primary classical texts of Ayurveda, the *Sushruta Samhita* and the *Charaka Samhita*, were penned much later, around 1000 B.C. The patron god Dhanwantari was, in fact, down the line in a succession of deities beginning with Brahma, whom Hindus regard as the creator. Dhanwantari, who according to mythology was a surgeon, descended from the Asvins, the divine physicians of paradise.

According to the principles of Ayurveda, each person is made up of a unique balance of three primary forces—or doshas—which interact on physical, psychological, and spiritual levels. These forces are called vata, pitta, and kapha. Vata is comprised of the elements air and space, and it's responsible for all motion and energy flow within the body. When vata is imbalanced, the result may be constipation, menstrual problems, poor digestion, and a restless or anxious mind. Pitta, comprised of fire and water, is responsible for metabolism, digestion, and energy production. When pitta is out of balance, one can become angry, digestion may suffer, and skin eruptions and ulcers may result. Kapha, comprised of earth and water, is responsible for the structure of the body. When kapha is out of balance, energy diminishes, enthusiasm wanes, and colds, flu, and congestion often result.

Since Ayurveda holds that disequilibrium among the three doshas results in diseases of various kinds, a patient is diagnosed not just according to the illness he or she may exhibit, but according to the condition of the doshas. Each person is typically dominant in one dosha. Thus a kapha-dominant patient with a cold and a pitta-dominant patient with a cold would be treated differently. In order to restore proper balance of the doshas and thus rebuild health, an Ayurvedic treatment plan will be tailored to the individual and will incorporate proper diet, exercise such as yoga, meditation, the use of specific medicinal herbal formulas, and any of several cleansing methods designed to rid the body of toxins. Health, according to this system, is not merely the absence of disease, but a dynamic state of harmony referred to as swastha. In this state, metabolic fire is strong, energy abundant, and the mind at peace.

We set off down the long, gloomy corridors of the Government Ayurvedic Medical College in the company of the head of Ayurvedic education at the college, a jovial and bright-spirited man introduced only as Dr. Lucas. We began by touring three different clinics that provide free health services to outpatients from the community. "This is our eye clinic," Dr. Lucas told us as we entered a series of connected rooms. "Here 60 to 80 people come every day for eye examinations, consultations, glasses, special vision-enhancing exercises, and Ayurvedic eye solutions made from herbal extracts. The doctors here specialize in treating cataracts and glaucoma, with very good success in many cases. We do not charge a fee for any of this work. It is all free to people in need."

In one room of the eye clinic, a small group of women sat reading fine print by candlelight. Reading small print without much light seemed counterintuitive to me, but Dr. Lucas said it was part of the series of exercises for maintaining fine vision in later life. "It protects the eyes from cataracts and glaucoma," he said. "Here we teach patients specific eye training exercises for 21 days. Then they practice on their own at home, coming back once every 2 weeks for a checkup. We offer a dozen eye exercises, plus treatments with medicated oils and Ayurvedic eye drops."

In another room, a woman practiced "swinging." She stood and swayed from left to right, while moving her gaze back and forth across a grate mounted on a stand that stood between her and a view of trees outside. "This is to loosen the eye muscles and reduce strain," Dr. Lucas pointed out. "These methods are so simple. Healing methods do not have to be complicated to be effective. I have practiced Ayurveda for a long time now, and I can tell you these exercises work. Many of these exercises have been used for thousands of years. They remove eye strain or help to correct vision problems, whether you are talking nearsightedness or farsightedness." On one table, neat rows of eyeglass lenses fit into slots in a large wooden case lined with felt. "So many people get glasses here," Dr. Lucas remarked, shaking his head with a satisfied smile.

At the clinic they also practice "palming"—rubbing the palms of the hands vigorously together and then placing them over the eyes. The fingers of one hand overlap those of the other over the forehead, and the palms are cupped in such a way as to deny all light to the eyes, which remain open and relaxed. Palming, which can be practiced sitting up or lying down, refreshes and comforts the eyes as it brightens sight. It's also a unique method of relaxation. If you practice palming at home, keep your hands cupped over your eyes for a minimum of 5 minutes.

The hospital allocates 225 of its 325 beds to those undergoing Ayurvedic treatment. The rest are for Unani, Siddha, yoga, and naturopathy patients. We walked down a long hallway, passing wards with worn beds and patients with various health problems. At the hospital's naturopathic clinic we were greeted by a radiant and alert young man named Satish, who explained the clinic's purpose. "Naturopathy involves the use of essentials from nature—such as food, water, rest, fresh air, and sunshine—to heal," he said. "We have gotten very good results again and again with these simple and natural methods." An average of 20 people per day are treated at the naturopathic clinic for such problems as chronic intestinal complaints, nerve disorders, paralysis, and various kinds of pain. "Sometimes we even get people who have had seizures and have not had success with any other form of treatment," Satish said. "Often they turn to us when other methods fail, and in many cases they recover."

The naturopathic clinic was equipped with an array of odd-looking bathtubs of varying shapes and sizes, and all of them colored in either pale green, aqua, or a fleshy pink. "Here we have many therapeutic baths, because we believe that hydrotherapy is one of the best forms of treatment for many ailments," Satish told us. An herb-infused steam bath compartment, used to treat respiratory disorders, was shaped like a truncated pyramid with a sitting bench inside and a hole on top for the patient's head to poke through. One tub looked like a low easy chair made of blue porcelain, with a central canal designed to accept the spine. A patient would lie recumbent on the apparatus, and jets in the canal would direct water at the spine at varying pressures and temperatures, depending on the diagnosis. "We use this mostly for neurological problems," Satish told us. The clinic also featured hip, foot, and arm baths, again for neurological problems, or pain. The hip bath was most often used for women with pelvic problems or digestive disorders.

"We also offer full colonic enemas to cleanse the bowels of impurities and to help restore vigor," Satish told me. "If you want, you could take a treatment." I politely declined the offer for intestinal irrigation, citing a pressing travel schedule. Satish rolled his head in a fluid figure eight, a universal and noncommittal Indian gesture signifying understanding. "Any time you want to come back, we will take good care of you."

The third clinic we visited offered traditional panchakarma treatment, a comprehensive rejuvenation treatment now offered in some Ayurvedic spas in the United States and Europe. Panchakarma treatment involves various types of massage and also offers internal cleansing techniques designed to rejuvenate the gastrointestinal tract as well as the mouth, nose, throat, and ear canals. A clean GI tract is considered especially paramount in Ayurvedic healing, following the proviso in the *Charaka Samhita* that "an unclean bowel is the root of all disease."

The panchakarma treatment tables at the Government Ayurvedic Medical College looked very much like the tables used by embalmers, with depressions to allow the various massage oils to run off. In one well-known panchakarma treatment, attendants pour warm sesame oil on the patient's forehead to induce a state of profound relaxation. (Thus the need for run-off canals.) In one room, Shahannah pointed to two women making oily compresses with a variety of powerfully aromatic herbs wrapped in cloth, and asked, "What are these for?" Dr. Lucas explained that the compresses would be employed to stimulate blood circulation and nerves during massages to help people recover from partial strokes and seizure disorders.

Dr. Lucas expounded on the benefits of panchakarma treatment, which include improved digestion, better absorption and assimilation of nutrients, deeper and more restful sleep, elimination of toxins, eradication of the "thought" of disease, promotion of longevity and rejuvenation through the rebuilding of body tissue, normalization of the menstrual cycle, increased awareness, increased emotional and mental clarity, and more physical flexibility. "And there is no question," Dr. Lucas said, "that panchakarma promotes deeper and more meaningful meditation by teaching us how to discover the seat of divinity within, thus creating a total balance of body, mind, and spirit."

I suggested that based on these benefits, everybody could probably use panchakarma treatment. With a knowing nod, Dr. Lucas said, "I can say that panchakarma is one of the great secrets of healthy living, and that all people can improve their health and longevity with these methods."

A MEDICINAL GARDEN

That afternoon, we cruised in Dr. Mitra's Nissan sedan across hot, dusty Bangalore to the Dhanwantari Vana herbal garden, a joint project of the awkwardly named Department of Indian System of Medicine and the Karnataka State Forest Department. A tall black statue of Dhanwantari stood on a pedestal of large stones. "This garden contains almost 500 species of medicinal plants," Dr. Paramesh informed us. More than 100 acres of medicinal plants, most of them identified with labels, gave vivid testimony to the effort being made in India to promote the use of these natural healers.

We came upon a large plot of *Gymnema sylvestre*, a plant known as the sugar destroyer. The plant is widely used in Ayurveda to regulate blood sugar in cases of adult diabetes. Gymnemic acid in the plant helps to regenerate pancreatic beta cells while curbing the craving for sweets. Near the *Gymnema* grew another widely used plant, *Adhatoda vasica*, also known as the Malabar nut. Containing an alkaloid called vasicine, plus vitamin C and carotenoids, *Adhatoda vasica* is regularly used in respiratory formulas. Close by we came upon *Tinospora cordifolia*, an immune system enhancer that contains tinosporine and other immunomodulating compounds, and that has been shown to boost the activity of protective macrophage cells.

Throughout the garden, bright red, yellow, and purple blossoms contrasted against the more profuse greens and earth tones. Shaded trellised walkways hung with creeping vines. Spears of soothing aloe vera thrust up from hundreds of red clay pots. Bees buzzed, dragonflies hovered, and birds sang in heavily foliated trees.

"We are seeing a great resurgence in Ayurveda," Dr. Mitra told us. "It has always been a very popular system, but now it is even more so. In fact, in India, Ayurvedic remedies outsell allopathic medicines by about four to one. Many celebrities are now touting the benefits of Ayurveda, and so it has become very much the in thing. Thus the demand for medicinal plants is at an all-time high."

As part of the promotion of medicinal plant cultivation, tens of thousands of seedlings stood in rows under shade trees.

"These seedlings are for growers," Dr. Paramesh said. "If you want to cultivate medicinal plants instead of just rice or cane or some other low-paying commodity, then you can come here and get all the seedlings you need. In this way, people are being encouraged to diversify their crops and to benefit economically by growing much-needed medicinal plants."

As we strolled through the Dhanwantari Vana project, we came upon an acre-size herbal garden with stones outlining the shape of a giant human body. Herbs were placed at locations of the body corresponding to their use. The brain enhancer gotu kola grew at the head, the herbal laxative senna was at the bowels, and anti-inflammatory plants like turmeric and boswellia thrived at the hip and knee joints. The garden was an ingenious teaching tool where one could quickly learn about the uses of more than two dozen herbs just by becoming familiar with their locations in the human-shaped garden.

As the broiling Indian sun rose like a cobra's head in the sky, fastidious Prakash and maniacal Prasad took us out into the countryside to an experimental medicinal plant farm run by the SAMI corporation, a maker of Ayurvedic herbal extracts. Prakash, who was generously on loan to us for our trip thanks to SAMI, made sure that we would see their agricultural work. In the company of herbal expert Suresh Kumar and former USDA agronomist Anil Chojar, we observed efforts to cultivate medicinal species from all over India.

In a large field, laborers broke up rich brown soil using

broad-bladed hoes, while the full intensity of south India's sweltering sun beat down upon their black backs. Wrapped only in waist cloths, the laborers directed water from a large standing pipe into newly cut irrigation channels. It appeared to be back-breaking work. "In India, there is very little mechanized farming," Anil Chojar commented. "Almost all cultivation of the soil and caring for crops is performed by hand. For most farmers, this is difficult subsistence farming. But with medicinal plants, even though the labor is very hard, there is a reward of greater profitability."

The purpose of the experimental farm, we learned, was to establish ways of cultivating medicinal plants from various regions of India, and even from other countries. "We will determine which cultivation methods work best for crops," explained Suresh Kumar, as we tramped through soft soil. "Once we are satisfied that we know how to produce large quantities of healthy plants, then we will share the information with local growers, some of whom we will contract to supply us with plant materials for extraction."

SAMI's goal was to eventually ensure an abundant supply of every major medicinal herb. We could see for ourselves ongoing successes and failures. Ashwagandha (*Withania somnifera*) grew well in the dark soil and oven-heat of the experimental farm. Aloe vera also appeared to do well. But echinacea, a major immune system–enhancing botanical that is popular in Europe and the United States, was faring poorly. Planted under shade cloth, the pink-petaled echinacea plants were bent and dying. Their stalks were withered, and several had turned black. Anil Chojar shook his head at the echinacea. "I think that maybe we will not be too successful with this particular herb, though there

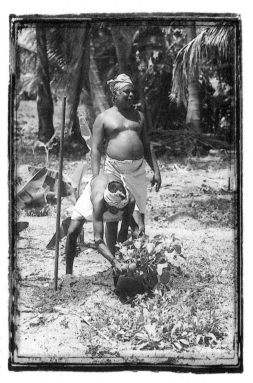

Digging fresh ashwagandha, the star of Ayurveda and India's most widely used medicinal plant

are some other methods we will try." To my eyes, echinacea looked like a plant that wouldn't be grown widely in the shimmering swelter of the south Indian plains.

One plant that appeared to be faring well was *Mucuna pruriens*. I reached out to touch a furry pod of the shrub, but Anil stopped me. "Don't do that," he warned. "It will give you a bad rash." So I inspected with caution a plant whose value is just being recognized outside the field of Ayurveda. *Mucuna* is a perennial shrub found wild throughout India, Sri Lanka, Southeast Asia, and Malaysia, from sea level up to 3,000 feet. Its fruit is a curved seed pod abundantly covered with bristles that apparently produce on contact the skin rash Anil had mentioned.

Commonly known as velvet bean or cowitch, *Mucuna pruriens* is primarily used in Ayurveda as a potent aphrodisiac drug capable of promoting semen production and increasing sexual vigor. *Mucuna* reputedly increases strength, and it is used therapeutically in cases of impotence, urinary disorders, leukorrhea, and spermatorrhea. In addition to its traditional uses, the plant has been shown to mitigate depression, enhance alertness, and improve coordination.

The seeds of the *Mucuna* pod contain lecithin, glucoside, and alkaloids such as nicotine, prurieninine, and prurienidine. Of especial interest is *Mucuna*'s content of L-dopa. Also known as levodopa, L-dopa is the naturally occurring form of the amino acid 3,4 dihydroxyphenylalanine, which is the precursor to the neurohormones norepinephrine and epinephrine, and of melanin, a pigment found in skin, hair, and the substantia nigra of the brain. In cases of Parkinson's disease, L-dopa is administered to alleviate rigidity as well as to slow movements and trembling, which result from a deficiency of dopamine in the brain. As research on *Mucuna pruriens* continues, the plant and its extracts will likely be more broadly used for brain enhancement. Increased demand will naturally require expanded cultivation.

I asked Anil Chojar if there was any single plant that stood to be an economic boon to growers. His answer: ashwagandha, or *Withania somnifera*. "There is not enough of it to satisfy demand, and it is used in at least half of all Ayurvedic preparations," he said. "There is not enough *Withania* in the wild, and at this point in time, growers are not cultivating enough acreage of this very valuable plant. We plan to grow a great deal of *Withania* ourselves and also to contract with a number of growers to produce it for us."

An Ayurvedic Aphrodisiac

Ashwagandha, India's most widely used medicinal plant, is often referred to as Indian ginseng and can be purchased in the United States. (See Resources on page 281 for information about specific brands of ashwagandha products.) Like ginseng in China, ashwagandha is thought to be useful in virtually all efforts to improve health, including sexual health. One Ayurvedic aphrodisiac formula uses ashwagandha this way:

1. Add 1 part ashwagandha to 10 parts milk and 1 part ghee (clarified butter).
2. Boil the mixture down until only the ghee apparently remains. This end product is called ashwagandha ghrita.
3. Take about a heaping tablespoon of this mixture in the morning and in the evening.

According to ancient texts, you will experience a significant boost in libido and sexual stamina. Does it work? Try it for yourself.

It's understandable that demand for ashwagandha is high. It can be used in any formula, for any purpose, with no known side effects. The root of the plant appears in remedies for cough, rheumatism, gynecological disorders, fatigue, emaciation, low libido, impotence, inflammatory conditions, ulcers, sore eyes, and diminished brain function. Ashwagandha is considered the most effective nerve tonic among all Ayurvedic herbs, and it's used widely for combating stress. Studies conducted in India show that the herb alleviates anxiety.

Can such broad uses for a single plant be legitimate? I'll answer that this way. Why would a huge body of people claim good results for so many health conditions over millennia if the plant weren't effective? What would be the incentive to carry a banner for an herb that doesn't work? According to every Ayurvedic text I have found, ashwagandha is the herbal jewel in the Ayurvedic crown, the plant that, above all others, can be used with at least some good effect in all cases, without exception.

What accounts for ashwagandha's remarkable healing versatility? The plant is rich in potent alkaloids, among which are withamosine, visamine, cuscohygrine, anahygrine, tropine, pseudotropine, anaferine, isopelletierine, and withaferin A. It contains a large number of novel compounds known as withanolides. Whether one or two of these compounds are responsible for the plant's beneficial health effects, or whether ashwagandha's value is due to an incredibly complex synergy of all its natural constituents, is a matter that may take a long time to solve by scientific means. But Ayurveda does not need to wait for science to "validate" a remedy that has proven itself for thousands of years. It is woven into the fabric of Indian medicine as surely as blue dye in jeans.

Adjacent to the SAMI experimental farm, an Indian peasant grew a few acres of rice and chile peppers. The paddy glistened an emerald green that shimmered in the hot breeze. The capsicum fruits of the chili plants were a bright red. The toothless farmer, wearing cracked glasses and clad in a lopsided turban and a grimy smock, greeted us with a welcoming smile and offered us tender coconut—a perfect refreshment in the blazing sun that we gladly accepted. The farmer and his helper crossed a field to climb a coconut tree and shake down some fruit, leaving us to admire the healthy chili-laden bushes. Once they returned, both men used long, rusty knives to deftly hack off the tops of the coconuts. When they handed them around, we saw that each coconut was brimming with nearly a pint of fresh, cool water, which we eagerly drank down. The farmer, though evidently very poor, would take no money for the coconuts, but he was happy to be photographed beside his proud work, a bumper crop of beautiful chile peppers nearly ready for market. When we departed, the farmer waved goodbye, turban perched lopsided on his head and bare toes dug into the soft soil of a farm made productive by months of hard labor in the blistering sun.

POTENT MEDICINE

Against the acoustic backdrop of Bangalore's morning roar, Shahannah and I ate a breakfast of chapatis, traditional flat bread made of whole wheat flour, with channa, curried chickpeas. "Do you think there's something wrong with this coffee?" Shahannah asked as she watched a small creamer worth of milk disappear into the blackness of her cup without changing the color of the liquid. "Mmm," I nodded. "They brewed it in the crankcase of a Tata truck." She gave up trying to modify the Stygian brew. We both opted for chai, India's mainstay beverage of black tea, milk, sugar, and spices.

Shahannah is accustomed to travel, as am I. Trained in environmental biology, she spent 3 years at sea in a turn-of-the-century Barcantine square rigger researching marine mammals. She's used to bad weather, cramped or dirty accommodations, poor facilities, bugs, bad transportation, and execrable coffee. In short, she's an ideal travel companion for a medicine hunter. True, our Ayurvedic research trip didn't require any time in the bush and was therefore reasonably comfortable, but other trips we've taken together have been far less so.

Shortly after breakfast, we climbed into the Tata Sumo—with wild Prasad at the wheel and fastidious Prakash riding shotgun—and dashed past lumbering elephants, steaming tea stalls, and bustling temples across busy Bangalore to the Government Ayurvedic Research Center. As we hurtled through intersections and accelerated blindly around tilting trucks and bulging buses, Prakash made motions with his hand as though patting the head of an unseen dog, uttering, "Slow, slow." His efforts appeared to have little impact on Prasad. "He has quit smoking," Prakash stated flatly, turning his head back toward us. "I have explained to him that smoking will lead him to an early grave, and so he has quit to save his life." Prasad, ever affable, nodded agreeably. "Next," Prakash announced, "I will get him to stop drinking. He drinks 180 milliliters of alcohol in the evenings. By the time our travels are over, Prasad will not be drinking." I had little doubt that the object of H. Prakash's reform efforts would change his ways.

At the research center, we met Dr. Yoganarasimhan, a botanist and author who has devoted his career to the study of medicinal plants in the state of Karnataka, of which Bangalore is the largest city. "In Karnataka, more than 1,200 species of plants are used in Ayurvedic preparations," Dr. Yoganarasimhan said as we sat in a drab corner of the center's cavernous herbarium. "Of these, only around 400 are used commonly." Work at the research center involves the proper plant identification as well as analysis to determine the chemical constituents. The herbarium contained cabinet after cabinet filled with meticulously stored, carefully identified botanical specimens. "Through this research we are increasing our knowledge of Ayurvedic medicines," he said. "And we are gaining a greater understanding of why the traditional preparations of this system of medicine are so effective."

When I asked if we could take photographs at the research center, Dr. Yoganarasimhan wagged his head sideways. "You would have to get permission from the directorate of government Ayurvedic programs," he told us. That office is in Delhi, at the opposite end of the subcontinent; it might as well have been on another planet. What's more, we would have to get permission from state officials as well. How long would all this take? "With luck, just a couple of months," Dr. Yoganarasimhan told me, adding optimistically, "You could begin to write letters now." In other words, in order to take a few simple photographs, we would have to scale a bureaucratic Everest against what I knew would be a howling blizzard of bureaucratic objection.

In contrast, the researchers at the Government Ayurvedic Research Center appeared to be engaged in valuable, innovative work. In a rudimentary lab filled with antique flasks and beakers and aged heaters, we met a Dr. Mary and a Dr. Shetey, who described their work to us. "First, we are analyzing each herb to determine its chemical profile," Dr. Mary told us. "We identify the characteristic constituents and the ratio in which they occur in the plant. Once we have completed this analysis, we try to identify the best ways to package traditional formulas to preserve their biological activity. After analyzing the herbs in a traditional formula, we prepare the formula according to instructions in the ancient Ayurvedic texts." The formulas then undergo stability tests, and eventually clinical trials. Finally, various storage methods are tried—brown glass containers, opaque plastic containers, and so on—to see how long the chemical constituents last under different conditions.

What it comes down to is that the research center is applying modern science to ancient formulas to establish quality standards, something that has become increasingly more important as Ayurvedic remedies are becoming more popular and, as a result, more widely distributed. An expert Ayurvedic practitioner working from scratch is likely to make a remedy correctly and administer it in the right doses. But what happens when traditional remedies become "products"? When they're marketed, distributed, and shipped far from where they were made? When they might sit on shelves for months at a time? As all of this occurs, issues of stability and potency inevitably arise. Like Sherlock Holmes and Dr. Watson, Dr. Shetey and Dr. Mary are working to resolve these thorny issues.

The research center is not all lab work. The herbarium there manufactures and distributes huge quantities of Ayurvedic medicines, which are distributed free to 50 clinics throughout Karnataka. The manufacturing facilities were a truly extraordinary spectacle—about as far removed from a modern pharmaceutical plant as can be imagined. An Ayurvedic specialist at the center called Dr. Prabhakan gave us a tour through the entire manufacturing process, beginning with vast storage rooms with high, vaulted ceilings, packed to the beams with hundreds of tons of cloth sacks groaning with dried, fragrant medicinal plants from all over Karnataka. "Every plant we need to make traditional formulas is here," he told us. "We are constantly buying plants and preparing them for medicines."

The first steps of herbal preparation are accomplished by chopping the plants with a short hand machete, and then putting them in what looked like huge dough mixers where large round stones attached to machine-driven belts whirl in a clockwise circle, grinding the plant material against the sides of the steel containers. Once the herbs are ground to the right fineness for whatever recipe they'll be used for, they are blended together in precise proportions. As I watched, women and men sat on the floor of a large hall covered with piles of herbs on cloths, weighing amounts on antique balance scales. The blended herbs, once weighed out, were placed in barrels for the next stages of preparation.

The Government Ayurvedic Research Center makes powdered herbal formulas, herbal pastes, herb-infused oils, concentrated herbal extracts, and formulas in a base of honey or jaggeree, an unrefined sugar. For each type of preparation, at least one large room is required. For alcohol-based herbal extracts, huge wooden casks 10 feet high stood on concrete platforms in neat rows. Filled with herbs and alcohol and sealed with mud, the casks sit for several months at a time until the stewing infusions in them are ready for bottling. I pressed an ear to the side of one huge cask and could hear a low bubbling sound, like digestion at work in deep, rumbling intestines.

In a large sooty room downstairs, workers in lunghis (loose cotton wraps) cooked herbs together with ghee (clarified butter) in giant cauldrons over roaring wood fires. The scene was out of the middle ages. Sweat glistened on the faces of the barefoot workers, and redness from the intense fire radiated off their bodies as they stirred mammoth pots with oarlike paddles. Giant stacks of wood gave evidence to the fuel requirements of this ancient process of herbal cookery. "This is very hard work," Dr. Prabhakan said. "These people are very dedicated." Shahannah and I received warm smiles from the workers and invitations to peer into the bubbling pots.

In the packing room, remedies of all types were put into containers by hand and then crated for shipment to free clinics. "This work is a service," Dr. Prabhakan told us with obvious pride. "We are doing this work for the good of suffering humanity. Most poor Indian people could not afford medicines. But they can go to clinics all over Karnataka and see doctors for free and receive the medicines they need, entirely without cost." The methods of manufacture may have been rudimentary, but the motives behind the manufacture of herbal formulas were noble. "If more people believed in helping others this way," Shahannah commented, "more people would stay well."

What a concept . . . a health system designed to help suffering humanity instead of HMOs oriented to the bottom line, cumbersome insurance companies who benefit nobody, and careless doctors who've long forgotten the real purpose of medicine. Our day at the Government Ayurvedic Research Center filled me with optimism that perhaps someday more health professionals would come to regard the practice of medicine as a service, not just a profit-driven enterprise.

THE CURCUMIN CURE

After a few days in Bangalore, Shahannah, Prakash, and I set off with Prasad driving in a southerly direction on the Old Mysore Highway—a rutted road in bad repair and barely two lanes wide. It was rush hour, a time of anarchy when the road was crammed with trucks, buses, cars, vans, bicycles, scooters, motorcycles, scooter cabs, oxcarts, tractors, cows, dogs, and children playing. Sari-clad women balanced huge loads on their heads. Men struggled to pedal bicycles hanging with hundreds of ripe coconuts or stacked impossibly high with brightly hued rubber pails, tubs, and basins. Horns blared, diesel smoke spewed from truck and bus tailpipes, drivers waved and shouted, and cows defecated on the road. Whole families were squeezed onto scooters.

Monstrous overloaded trucks barreled heedlessly through a sea of people, animals, and smaller vehicles, swathing them in dust and diesel fumes. They bore down on us like riders from hell, with the brands Tata and Ashok Leyland in large letters on their grills, their windows festooned with glitter, tinsel, and pictures of deities. Elaborate paint jobs on the sides of trucks depicted the play of the gods in scenes from Hindu scriptures. During our trip, I would dream at night of giant truck grills with ominous headlights rushing at me in the dark. Daredevil Prasad, gripping the wheel intensely, double-passed buses passing trucks, against oncoming double-passers, in an endless game of chicken. Prakash vainly employed his downward patting motion—"slow, slow"—as we screamed down the road.

India is a land of temples large and small, and many of them are found conveniently by the roadsides. As we motored along the Old Mysore Highway, we passed small shrines on sidewalks, multi-deity spires rising a hundred feet, and imposing single gods rising one or two stories above temple rooftops. Temple bells clanged, dhoti-clad priests performed ceremonies to propitiate the gods, and bustling streams of devotees came and went. Brahma, Vishnu, Siva, Arjuna, Krishna, Indra, Hanuman, Ganesh, Nandi, Parvati, Kali, Lakshmi, and dozens of other multicolored gods and goddesses graced walls and roofs. Speakers hanging from trees and posts blasted holy music at ear-splitting volume. Vendors sold bells, incense, marigold blossoms, candles, pictures of deities, posters, bangles, beads, dashboard ornaments, sweets, tea, soda, ice cream, water coconuts, incense burners, scented oils, and statues of favorite gods. In India, the god business is very good business indeed. As we had seen at Prakash's home, almost every Indian household maintains a small shrine for the performance of daily ceremonies, which require many or most of the wares sold by temple vendors.

After eating dust for hours, we arrived alive at the SAMI corporation's curcumin extraction facility in the city of Mysore. There we met the general manager of operations, Karunakar Narayan, who mentioned that he attended Benares Hindu University right about the time that Allen Ginsburg was there in the 1960s. This led to a general discussion of that era, with Karunakar wondering aloud if any of those experiences made a difference. Shahannah said, "Those times fashioned us into what we are today."

At the laboratory we met two chemists who specialize in extracting useful resins from oil-bearing plants of all kinds. They showed us samples of clove oil, cardamom oil, cinnamon oil, ginger oil, and their specialty, the oleoresin of turmeric root. It's turmeric root that imparts the yellow to curries and that yields the medicinally valuable compound called curcumin, an anti-inflammatory agent that holds promise for the relief and treatment of arthritis. There were at least 10 different varieties of turmeric (*Curcuma longa*) at the lab. Some were slender and dark, others chubby and orange. "The variations in these roots have to do with soil conditions and altitude," one of the chemists told us. "The best varieties of turmeric yield the highest levels of curcumin, about 3 percent by weight."

The extraction facility—powered by boilers stoked with great lengths of wood—processes about 1,000 tons of turmeric each year for a total annual yield of 35 tons of curcumin extract, all of which is shipped to the United States for use in dietary supplements. Dried turmeric root is fed by hand into a large, belt-driven mechanical grinder that powders the root and then

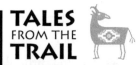

TALES
FROM THE
TRAIL

Currying Favor with Your Health

The more we learn about the aromatic herbs and spices in an Indian masala, or curry, the more we discover the clever medicine behind these time-honored seasonings. One of these is the curcumin extracted from the turmeric root.

Curcumin supplements are valuable to health and are available in health food stores. But you can also get curcumin by eating spices made from the turmeric root. Since turmeric is a food, it's a better choice. My favorite method of enjoying turmeric is simply making lots of great-tasting yellow curries.

Use ground turmeric cooked in hot oil as your base for a homemade curry sauce that you can use with just about any dish. Also include garlic, hot chile peppers, some cardamom, cumin, a bit of cinnamon, black pepper, a touch of clove—and any other spices you like.

blows it into a containment vessel. Modern stainless steel extraction tanks containing tons of raw, dried turmeric root powder are filled with acetone to extract the curcumin. The acetone runs through the powdered turmeric root and then out the bottom of the extraction tank. It may be poured in through the top as many as seven times, until the fluid runs clear. Then the fluid is percolated, evaporating the acetone and leaving a thick, gooey oleoresin. This resin is put into large ovens where it hardens into cakes, which in turn are ground into the powder used in herbal formulas.

A staple medicine in the millennia-old Ayurvedic system, turmeric is cultivated throughout tropical regions of Asia. Its medicinal value is the subject of much serious research. An Indian double-blind clinical trial involving patients with rheumatoid arthritis found that administration of oral doses of curcumin offered significant relief from morning stiffness, walking difficulties, joint swelling, and general pain and discomfort. In other arthritis studies performed with rats and pigeons, curcumin demonstrated significant anti-inflammatory activity. Studies conducted at the Central Drug Research Institute in Lucknow, India, found that curcumin is an effective nonsteroidal anti-inflammatory, though it must be consumed in larger quantities than many other anti-inflammatory drugs. Curcumin appears to offer pulmonary benefits as well. Patients with respiratory diseases who were treated with curcumin experienced varying degrees of relief from coughing, excessive sputum, and labored breathing.

In vitro studies performed in India and Japan show that curcumin may help protect the heart. In rat studies, curcumin decreased liver cholesterol, increased fecal excretion of cholesterol, and lowered serum cholesterol. Rats fed curcumin had one-half to one-third the serum and liver cholesterol levels of rats that were not fed curcumin. In still other animal studies, curcumin inhibited the growth of ovarian cancer cells.

In one study, curcumin ointment reduced itching and pain from external cancerous lesions in 90 percent of cases. Other studies on wound-healing showed that topically applied curcumin accelerates the healing of infected and noninfected wounds.

Curcumin also suppresses the growth of some pathogenic, food-borne bacteria, which probably accounts for its widespread use in cultures where refrigeration is a rarity. And studies show that curcumin protects liver cells against potent toxins, including carbon tetrachloride.

After touring the curcumin extraction facility, we met a Dr. Kalyanaraman, who is a chemist with an extensive background in both Ayurveda and state-of-the-art extraction science. Dr. Kalyanaraman told us of his success in creating a potent anti-dysentery medicine from the simplest ingredients, made right at the bench of his laboratory. It seems that a few years back, he was attending a medical conference right there in Mysore when several of the Western physicians in attendance became sick with diarrhea. "I gave them a blend of the oleoresins of ginger, black pepper, and turmeric, and I promised that they would get better soon," he said. "Frankly, I don't think they believed me, but they were in pitiful condition, so they tried my remedy. Within 24 hours of first taking the formula, all the doctors who had fallen ill were back on their feet and recovered from the diarrhea. Do you know, they were so surprised." Dr. Kalyanaraman shook his head and chuckled, recalling how surprised the Western doctors were. "Nature yields truly miraculous healing ingredients," he said. "We do not need to make up anything synthetic. We can find whatever we require in the marvelous chemistry of plants."

Outside Mysore, Chamundi Hill rises high above the shimmering, dusty plains, a grand imposition upon the landscape, much like Australia's Ayer's Rock or Georgia's Stone Mountain. At the very top of the hill sits the grand Sri Chamundeshwari temple, named after the protective god who, legend has it, saved the people of that area from the wrathful rampages of the buffalo-headed demon Mahishasura. Inside the cool, high-ceilinged marble halls of the temple, a group of priests made continual offerings of fruit, flowers, and fire to a statue of Chamundeshwari, which stood in a gilded inner sanctum with garlands of flowers around its neck. Shahannah and I gave offerings of rupees for the temple, and in return received handfuls of flower blossoms and had our foreheads smeared with chandan, a sacred paste of ground sandalwood. Chattering monkeys scampered about, snatching biscuits from unsuspecting temple visitors, leaping from railings to bells to standing sculptures, and scaling the steep, ornately carved outer temple walls.

One thousand steps downhill from the temple, we visited the colossal 16-foot high statue of the bull-god Nandi, the celestial mount of Siva, who is widely considered the most powerful in the pantheon of Hindu gods and is the lord and protector of yogis and mystics. Nandi, carved in the 17th century out of a single boulder, was seated regally atop a great stone platform with a carved bell around his neck and anklets above each hoof. The statue, which commands a spectacular view of the Mysore plains, appeared imbued with real life. He looked like he could rise at any moment.

Behind the giant statue of Nandi, a small sign indicated a cave temple dedicated to the god Siva. Outside the entrance, attendants swept the ground, lit incense, and performed the ongoing chores of a busy holy site. Crouching, we crabbed through the low entrance into a small cave not 4 feet high. Inside, a sparkling blue ceramic-tiled floor and walls surrounded an ornate altar with statues of Siva, photographs of some of India's great saints, smoking incense, flickering votive candles, brilliant flowers, and a bucket of rock sugar. Holy music played from a cassette machine. A slender yogi dressed in a red dhoti and a loose-fitting shirt, called a kurta, greeted us from where he was sitting at a corner of the altar. He had long hair and bright eyes, and inquired in impeccable English where we were from. "Boston," I told him. He gave a knowing nod. "Ah, Boston Tea Party." Shahannah and I both laughed at the unexpected reference.

He was Jamnagar Yogi, the ascetic in the Siva cave temple who had traveled the Himalayan mountain region for several years, visiting pilgrimage sites and meeting great saints. "But you know, it was just too cold," he laughed. "I eventually thought that it was better to head back to the south. So I came here, and now I have settled in this temple, and you will always find me here. I can serve people very well here and can remember God, and I don't have to freeze." He gave the carefree laugh of a man for whom life's troubles are trifling matters.

After some more chatting, Jamnagar asked us if we would care for some tea. We readily accepted. Jamnagar squatted beside a small gas burner, atop of which he placed a pot filled with water. We watched him make the tea with full and happy attention as though it were his sole function in the world, and his greatest delight. When he was finished, he handed each of us a hot stainless steel cup of absolutely perfect tea. "We will have a Chamundi Tea Party," he quipped. Jamnagar laughed and we laughed, and we all drank tea with carefree hearts and listened to holy music on the cassette, while outside the day grew dim and the last orange light of the Indian sun retreated across the arid plains and disappeared behind a soft haze of dust.

COCA-COLA
AYURVEDA

Ayurveda's renaissance is reverberating beyond India's borders, as people in all countries become increasingly attracted to this ancient system of plant-based medicines and therapies. Ayurvedic philosophy is brilliantly summed up in a phrase from an ancient text: "May all be happy, may all be healthy, may all experience that which is good, and let no one suffer." That philosophy was vindicated many times over as we continued our investigation of Ayurveda as it's actually practiced in the land of its origins.

In the shadow of great Chamundi Hill, Shahannah and I found ourselves at the Indus Valley Ayurvedic Center (IVAC), a modern Ayurvedic retreat that offers all of the traditional therapies of Ayurveda with unsurpassed modern amenities and attention to detail. India's Ayurvedic treatment centers run from the wholly ghastly to the sublime. Some Ayurvedic clinics and spas are so filthy, unsanitary, and run-down as to be truly scary. But this one, highly recommended to us by our friend Dr. Raj Bammi back in Bangalore, was deep into the realm of the sublime.

"What a perfect time for you to arrive," Dr. Krishna beamed, greeting us with warm handshakes and soulful eye contact. "We are just about to plant the very first tree in our medicinal garden. We have picked this day, and this exact time, as most auspicious according to astrology. And now you show up at this exact moment. This is clearly more than coincidence. I think it is divine providence. Everything happens for a reason in the grand order of things, don't you think? Please come with us to the planting ceremony."

About a mile down the road from the high, whitewashed walls of the IVAC front entrance, we stood in a field with co-founders Dr. Talavane Krishna and his wife, Anita. As the sun of the Mysore plains cooked us, the priest performed a planting ceremony for a small tree in the northeast corner of a field. "Energetically speaking, this is the very best place for the planting of this first tree, according to the ancient principles of vaastu," explained Dr. Krishna, who is also the center's director.

After the ceremony, we sat on the veranda of the IVAC main building, shaded by a broad green awning. In marked contrast to the loud, dusty, tumultuous streets we'd been driving, IVAC offered a pervasive sense of ease. "The effect that people experience here," Dr. Krishna said, "is a result of the vaastu of this place." He likened vaastu to the ancient Chinese system of Feng Shui, but older and more accurate. "In vaastu, the careful placement and order of things facilitates a balanced flow of energy," he went on. "And this promotes harmony and good fortune. We have taken extraordinary pains to make sure that everything conforms to the life-enhancing principles of vaastu, and that the environment is peaceful and harmonious."

It was evident from our conversation that Dr. Krishna and Anita have delved deeply and enthusiastically into the vaastu system. That included positioning the rooms, fountains, shade trees—all aspects of the IVAC facilities—for a powerful harmony. The Krishnas even provide consultation to others who literally need to get their houses in order. "We have been to homes," Anita told us, "where the entrance was in the wrong place, where beds were all facing the wrong direction, and the people living there had problems like sickness or misfortune." Dr. Krishna finished, "But then once we helped the people to correct a few simple things, and to rearrange the vaastu of their homes, their lives changed for the better." I'd heard stranger tales, and I certainly didn't discount the notion that rearranging a home could make a difference in the attitude and experience of the people living there. Whether or not proper vaastu was the wellspring of harmony at IVAC, the peace and serenity there were undeniable.

We entered the main building, with its cool, gently circulating air and clean marble floors. Pale blue light bathed the mezzanine in the main hall. I believe that everyone I know, however fussy, could immediately appreciate this place. "You know, almost everybody has said that this place feels like a temple," Dr. Krishna commented. "We are so happy for that. We want that kind of serenity."

Our tour of IVAC reminded me of *Lifestyles of the Rich and Famous*. Clearly what was being offered here was Ayurveda for the well-heeled. One treatment session we would try later would cost more than $90 in United States currency, well beyond the reach of India's huddled masses. Dr. Krishna led us from one room to the next, commenting on the attention to detail that had gone into planning everything from door trim to the construction of beds. Treatment rooms for IVAC's special

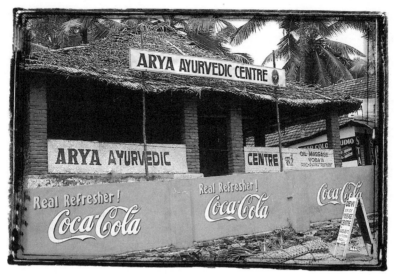

Ayurveda in India: as popular as Coca-Cola

therapies included gleaming modern conveniences. Plumbing, which can be a nightmare in India, was in impeccable working order. Guest rooms were exquisitely appointed with one-of-a-kind handcrafted furniture designed by Dr. Krishna. Tables, chairs, beds, massage tables, bathrooms, lighting, and decorations were carved out of exotic woods and polished to a lustrous beauty that revealed sumptuous grains. Standing in one room, plainly proud of his handiwork, Dr. Krishna announced, "You see, Ayurveda is all the rage now. It is as popular as, well, Coca-Cola! So we decided to create a place that even the fussiest clients like Madonna would come to." I suggested that Madonna might want 24-hour room service. "We would simply explain that we do not offer that," replied Dr. Krishna, clearly king of this castle.

An anesthesiologist who practiced medicine for more than 20 years in the West, Dr. Krishna understands what is required to run a health facility. A team of expert Ayurvedic physicians meets the health needs of all IVAC guests, each of whom fills out a detailed health questionnaire and undergoes a basic medical exam. On the basis of this examination, various courses of therapy are recommended. "We approach every person according to the traditional diagnosis of the doshas," said Dr. Krishna. "But we also pay attention to conditions that can be understood by Western methods of diagnosis. We try to be as thorough as possible, to be correct in our recommendations, and to put our guests at ease."

Some people go to IVAC purely for rejuvenation—for a good cleansing, invigorating massages, and yoga and meditation. Others go for more serious health conditions, including digestive complaints, obesity, circulatory problems, and neurological disorders. Each of these needs has a specific Ayurvedic therapy. "Did you know," Anita Krishna asked, "that some of the Ayurvedic massage methods actually get rid of cellulite?" Dr. Krishna concurred, describing how the intense circulation-enhancing effect of certain Ayurvedic massages seems to break up the fatty deposits of cellulite, restoring tone and luster to formerly lumpy, fatty skin. Shahannah suggested that an effective cellulite treatment alone could keep IVAC booked forever. Dr. Krishna nodded. "Cellulite absolutely goes away with these massages," he said. "It is not difficult. Ayurveda has an answer for every problem."

For those who are not seasoned Asian travelers, the strange tastes and frequent poor hygiene involved with Indian food can cause problems. In this regard, we found IVAC a welcome way station for the wary palate. We toured a large, spotless kitchen with a team of cooks using ultra-purified water and sparkling modern appliances. When we broke for lunch, Shahannah and I were delightfully surprised by the exquisite quality of the food. "When people undergo cleansing or some kind of treatment, often food is one of their few comforts," Dr. Krishna said. "So of course it must be the finest quality and best tasting."

Later, we relaxed in the Krishnas' spectacular home with cups of heavenly coffee. "You would be surprised how much trouble we put into making even a simple cup of coffee," Dr. Krishna said with enthusiasm. "I select the green beans myself. Did I tell you that my family owns a coffee plantation? Then I make sure that the beans are roasted exactly to perfection. And also you must grind them properly, neither too coarse nor too fine, and use the right quantity of freshly ground coffee for each cup, and use fresh, cold water." Dr. Krishna was increasingly animated as he described the fanatic's path to perfect coffee. "It is really a science, if you want to get right down to it," he said. "But I think all the trouble is worth it." After being thoroughly disappointed by Indian coffee, which ran from boiled, bitter brews to hideous Nescafé, we agreed. Dr. Krishna's coffee was unquestionably the perfect cup.

Conversation is fine, but Shahannah and I were ready to lay our bodies down and sample Ayurvedic treatments for ourselves. The next morning we awoke early and headed over from our shabby hotel in Mysore to IVAC for scheduled sessions of abhyanga, a special therapeutic massage method of panchakarma, Ayurveda's famous restorative treatment program.

We arrived at the center at 7:30 A.M. and were met by medical doctors on the IVAC staff. They gave us each basic physical exams and went through detailed medical questionnaires, asking us about our respective medical histories, medications, past surgeries, and current problems. Shahannah and I accounted for our various accidents and surgeries, but we could offer no current use of medication or health problems.

I was first for abhyanga, and I was eager. I was ushered into a serene therapy room, the centerpiece of which was an exquisite, handcrafted African teak massage table with carved, oil-catching channels. Soft sitar music played over clear speakers. The sweet scent of champa incense danced lightly in the air. The temperature was perfect. I was provided with a very brief loincloth in place of my shorts and shirt. Once in the loincloth I remarked to myself what a nifty item of clothing it was for such a hot climate. Too bad loincloths are discouraged in modern society.

For the first part of the massage, I was seated in a comfortable chair. Two masseurs dressed in crisp white jackets initiated the session by putting their hands together solemnly in prayer and chanting a long mantra intended to invoke cosmic healing powers. After the divine invocation, the two men poured herb-infused sesame oil onto the top of my head and began to massage my entire head, face, and neck in perfect synchrony, one working on the left and the other on the right. I noted to myself that the oil contained camphor, which served to open and refresh my sinuses and ear canals as I slipped into a gentle state of complete calm.

After several minutes of thorough head-and-shoulder massage, I was invited to lie on the table. The two masseurs poured oil all over me, and again in perfect synchrony began to massage virtually every inch of my body. Keeping a constant oil stream going, for maximum lubrication and topical herbal medication, they each worked on the same part of my body, one on the left, one on the right, with equal pressure. This exquisite massage, which seemed to open every pore and loosen every sinew, went on for a full hour. Once the two masseurs were done, I thought I was, too. As it turned out, the two-man massage was just the warm-up act for the main event.

With a silent flurry of white jackets and silken saris, two more men and two women then entered the treatment room. The women set up a gas burner, upon which they placed a pot filled with a mixture of hot, medicated oil and milk. Into this simmering concoction they dipped cloth bags filled with special red rice. Once the bags were thoroughly soaked, each of the four men took one in hand, and then they all began to rub my body vigorously with the hot, gooey, aromatic rice bags, sending me into absolute ecstasy. Employing the same extraordinary symmetry, but this time in perfectly articulated four-part harmony, they vigorously rubbed and re-rubbed every part of my mortal frame. Every few minutes the women re-dipped the cloth bags into the hot medicated milk and oil concoction. As the massage progressed, I was slathered in hot, milky goo.

No massage or body therapy I've ever received rivaled the glorious experience of being massaged for a full hour by the four experts with the dripping rice bags. Sure, it sounds strange as hell. But the treatment is one of those rare Ayurvedic jewels refined and perfected over millennia. When the whole session was over, I felt as though I had been meditating for a few weeks. All tension in my body was gone. My mind was clear and calm, and I felt like a lotus upon an ocean of bliss.

Shahannah floated out of her abhyanga treatment revitalized and beatific. We looked at each other and burst out laughing, filled with pure joy. "Many people undergo this course of treatment every day for 1 or 2 weeks," Dr. Krishna told us over tea. "In some cases they might even take a month's course." I laughed out loud trying to imagine that extraordinary treatment every day for a week or a month. Perhaps Ayurveda, as some advocates suggest, really is a path to enlightenment.

THE COOL BLUE HILLS

With Prasad at the wheel, we made our way out of the baking, brown-dusty Mysore plains, passing from the state of Karnataka into the state of Tamil Nadu. As we rode, we enjoyed the vast, picturesque forests of the Bandipur and Mudumalai Wildlife Sanctuaries, where we espied sambar and forest elephants. In the Bandipur sanctuary, trekking routes were shut down as a result of the activities of one man, a brigand named Veerappan, who has killed park officers and elephants and is known as a smuggler of ivory and sandalwood. Signs on the road advised motorists to stay in their cars in the event of elephant sightings. This was a wise recommendation. An angry elephant can quickly turn a car into a tangled heap of scrap metal.

After several hours of driving, we began to climb into the Nilgiri Hills, passing through large, fragrant stands of blue eucalyptus trees, whose invigorating scent drenched the air. Also known as the Blue Mountains, the Nilgiris are the second oldest mountain range in India, after the Himalayas. The Nilgiri Hills cover 2,542 square miles of hills, forests, and lakes, with a high point, Dodabetta Peak, of just over 8,500 feet. These mountains afford scenic views and host lush tea plantations and aromatic eucalyptus groves. Also, due to a temperate climate, twice-yearly monsoons, and their varying altitudes, the Nilgiri Hills offer rich and diverse flora.

As a heavy rain began to fall, we arrived in Ooty, site of the first of the Indian hill stations, a cottage-filled enclave established by the British to escape the suffocating heat of the plains during summer. Our primary destination in Ooty was the JSS College of Pharmacy, where researchers are fulfilling the difficult task of chronicling the medicinal plant use of small groups of tribal natives. In doing so, they have created one of the most distinguished repositories of medicinal plant information in India.

In the Nilgiris, five tribal groups still live separate and distinct from the rest of integrated Indian society. The Todas, Kotas, Kurumbas, Irulas, and Paniyas are virtually unknown outside of India—and little known within it. With a combined population of approximately 20,000, these groups are small. Medicine experts among the Nilgiri tribes possess broad knowledge of the plants in the hills and their medicinal uses. These individuals, known as madhukara, are similar to the shamans of the Amazon rain forest in their breadth of medicinal knowledge. Thus they are profound resources.

"We have spent many years working among the madhukara," explained a cheerful Dr. Subbaraju, who as head of the JSS department of pharmacognosy heads up investigation into traditional medicinal uses of the region's plants as well as their chemical constituents and their biological activity. "This work is very important to us, and we have made strong progress in preserving much of this valuable plant knowledge."

Dr. Subbaraju's manner was so mild and humble that it would be easy to underestimate the profound nature of the

Ayurveda in the U.S.A.

In the United States, you'll usually find single Ayurvedic herbs, such as *Gymnema* or ashwagandha, in capsules. You may also be able to find formulas for specific health purposes, such as laxatives or arthritis pain relievers. One American twist is that manufacturers are not allowed to explicitly state that formulas are for the relief of a specific health problem. You'll find that they skirt the ban by using names like "ArthroVeda." Not hard to figure out, is it?

Natural food stores and Indian specialty stores are your best sources for Ayurvedic herbs in the United States. In Resources on page 281, I give some recommendations. In stores where Ayurvedic remedies are sold, you may find books that describe various Ayurvedic herbs and their uses.

Actual Ayurvedic treatment, though it can be found in the United States, is more problematic. You should choose only a practitioner trained and certified in India. There are numerous self-styled Ayurvedic "experts" who advertise in some New Age and alternative publications, but I would not trust their expertise. Ayurveda is a serious pursuit requiring in-depth education and expertise. Just as you would want only a licensed dentist to drill your teeth, only a thoroughly trained Ayurvedic physician will suffice.

Though true Ayurvedic experts are available, they're mostly concentrated on the West and East Coasts. Outside of the Los Angeles, San Francisco, New York, and Boston areas, you won't find many.

work he was describing. In fact, JSS has undertaken a mammoth task, and successfully so. Already the college has identified 300 indigenous medicinal plants, along with their correct botanical names and parts used. In addition, Dr. Subbaraju's team has analyzed the chemical constituents of many of these plants, and has conducted extensive studies on their biological activity.

In many instances, the plants used among the hill tribes of the Nilgiri region are the same as those employed in the three traditional systems of Indian medicine—Ayurveda, Siddha, and Unani. But some are unique to that region. The library at JSS College of Pharmacy contains hundreds of volumes on regional medicinal plants and their uses. Many of the herbal formulas used by the Nilgiri tribespeople have been studied in-depth, and they are the subjects of entire works published by the college. Some of the more valuable formulas chronicled in this way may eventually be developed as botanical products for the world supplement market.

The scientists at JSS College of Pharmacy told us they have been astounded by the sophisticated understanding of the tribal peoples. For example, the tribal people boil some herbs in buffalo milk rather than cow's milk to make medicines. They had discovered what chemists knew only after modern analysis— that certain herbs contain fat-soluble active compounds, which are extracted far more efficiently with fatty buffalo milk than with less-fatty cow's milk. "We have also discovered that the tribal people have figured out certain methods of time release for particular herbs," Dr. Subbaraju told us. "Actually, their understanding of plants and how they work is quite profound. Most important, they know how to heal a great many ailments."

Another tribal combination herbal remedy has proved very effective as an anti-diabetic formula, and it's now undergoing development at JSS College of Pharmacy as a medicine. It contains *Gymnema sylvestre*, Ayurveda's famed herb for controlling blood sugar, plus three other effective anti-diabetic herbs unique to the tribes: *Syzygirim cumiri*, *Cassia ariculata*, and *Prunus amygdalus*.

A couple of days after our first visit to the college, Shahannah and I made our way to a Toda village set on a hilltop on the edge of Ooty, beside giant eucalyptus trees. There we sat with a priest and guide named B. Inbaraj. "Many Toda have moved away into towns," he told us. "But many have also stayed, because our way of life is different from the life of other Indians. Everybody here"—he swept his hand to include the whole village—"is Toda."

We asked B. Inbaraj about medicinal plants. "We have too many," he told us, pursing his lips. "Almost every plant can be used for something. But some are especially helpful. Do you know we have plants that can prevent death from a cobra bite? Yes, it is true. We have all used these. We've also used plants for bad cuts, to make the skin heal quickly, and for broken bones. In these hills there are no hospitals. We must be the doctors. So we take the necessary plants from nature, and we use them. We cannot cure everything, but most problems we can fix."

While I took notes, Inbaraj discussed a number of plants and their uses. "Sometimes you get excited too much, and you need to calm down. You can take the flowers of kungumappu (*Crocus sativus*). Or if you want to make more sex, we use tutti (*Abutilon indicum*), the seeds and root. Even for cancer. You know cancer? We use the leaves and roots of kattamanaku (*Jatropa curcas*). If you take that, many times cancer will go away." He mentioned three plants for snake bites: amman pacharisi (*Euphorbia hirta*), aattalaree (*Polygonum glabrum*), and pavali (*Thphorsiap urporea*). "You see, we must have many plants for snakebites," he said, "because we have many snakes."

The conversation with B. Inbaraj went on for a long time. "I can take you out into the mountains; you will see so many plants," he said. Then he added, "Snakes, too." He took us over to a Quonset-hut–shaped building of thick mud brick, with a heavy roof of thatched grass tightly knotted and tied down. On the front of the building, ancient glyphs portrayed the sun, moon, man, and woman. "This is our temple," Inbaraj told us. "I am a priest, so I come here and make ceremony. When I do that, I don't drink alcohol. But other times, I drink." He led us around to the back of the small temple. About 2 feet off the ground, a small square hole was cut out of the mud brick. "Every morning at about 6:30, a large cobra snake comes into the temple through here," he said. "We give him a plate of milk. He drinks the whole thing and never hurts anybody. He is very, very peaceful. And big. Then when he is full, he goes out. Every day."

Set atop a high hill, commanding a fine view of the beautiful Nilgiris, the Toda village stood apart from mainstream Indian hill culture, existing in a different time, when bizarre glyphs were the signs of the day and snakes were welcome, well-fed guests in temples.

HILLS OF TEA

Zooming east out of Ooty on a breezy, sunny day along winding mountain roads and steep, narrow grades, our happy quartet set course for the hills of Coonoor. I was eager to see the tea plantations there, and the majestic plantations of Coonoor in the Nilgiri Hills did not disappoint. They were even more beautiful than I had imagined. Shahannah and I were reminded of the Amazon, with its innumerable shades of green. Stands of blue-green shady eucalyptus trees lined the roads, and the verdant plantations glistened in the sun. Made from the leaves of *Camellia sinensis*, tea is the second most commonly drunk beverage in the world, after water. Some teas are considered truly superb, like very fine wines. The plantations of Coonoor provide some of the finest, most delicately fragrant tea in the world.

The plantations went on for dozens of miles over high, beautiful hills. At the different plantations, we saw workers—exclusively women—picking tea leaves with fast, nimble fingers and putting them into large cloth bags. I walked way into the chest-high tea bushes to watch the picking up close. Dexterity is essential for the task, since the picking or "plucking" of tea determines to a great extent the fineness of the tea. A skilled plucker will expertly race practiced fingers over the top of a tea bush, plucking only the topmost, youngest leaves, snapping the stems with a quick twist of the fingers. Throughout all of the plantations, we saw hundreds of women picking tea, and most of them were gracious about allowing us to take their photographs. We spent the entire day walking through plantations, admiring the plants and the women who carefully harvested the tea leaves.

All tea starts out as green tea. When fresh, tender tea leaves are picked, you get green tea by drying the leaves straightaway. To make black tea, the tender green leaves of the tea bush must be picked, fermented, and then dried. While any color of tea is beneficial to health, scientists have found that green tea especially is one of the most beneficial beverages in the world. A common beverage drunk widely throughout Asia, green tea holds great promise as a source of potent medicinal compounds.

In particular, green tea contains a family of antioxidant compounds known as polyphenols. There are four primary polyphenols in green tea—epicatechin (EC), epicatechin gallate (ECG), epigallocatechin (EGC), and epigallocatechin gallate (EGCg). While all four catechins appear to possess medicinal value, EGCg occurs in the greatest concentration and appears to offer the strongest antioxidant benefits. EGCg is appreciably more potent an antioxidant than vitamin E.

Green tea appears to protect the heart. It lowers cholesterol by inhibiting cholesterol absorption and reducing the body's cholesterol production. Green tea also reduces blood pressure by inhibiting the ACE enzyme, or angiotensin converting enzyme. This is the same mechanism by which several expensive prescription blood pressure medicines work. In addition, green tea reduces blood platelet stickiness, thus lowering the risk of atherosclerosis, or hardening of the arteries. A study reported by Japan's National Defense Medical College found that serum cholesterol levels were inversely related to green tea consumption. In other words, the more green tea you drink, the lower your cholesterol level. Black tea also plays a role in maintaining a healthy heart. A study of approximately 20,000 adults conducted in Oppland County, Norway, showed that the con-

The magnificent tea plantations of Coonoor

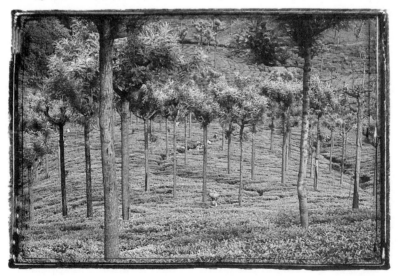

sumption of black tea lowered cholesterol, reduced blood pressure, and decreased the risk of coronary disease.

On the cancer front, the news about green tea is even more promising. Researchers at the Fourth Chemical Congress of North America reported that in animal studies, green tea helped to prevent tumors of the lung, liver, skin, and digestive tract. A paper published by the University Hospitals of Cleveland and Case Western Reserve University described the antimutagenic and anticarcinogenic effects of green tea polyphenols (GTP). These polyphenols inhibit the P450 enzyme system in the liver, which is responsible for the production of carcinogens. Green tea also inhibits the mutagenic effects of a variety of extremely potent toxins, including aflatoxin, salmonella typhimurium, a methanol extract of coal tar, and several others.

Japanese studies conducted at Okayama University show that green tea polyphenols lower the risk of cancer by preventing genetic damage from bacterial and chemical carcinogens. A Japanese National Cancer Center Research Institute study concluded that epigallocatechin gallate (EGCg) from green tea had multidimensional anticancer activity. EGCg inhibited tumor production, suppressed free radical formation, and reduced the overall risk of cancer. A toxicology study at the Indiana University School of Medicine found that green tea extract inhibited the formation of liver cancer. Other research, conducted at the British Columbia Cancer Research Center, indicated that the simultaneous consumption of green tea with certain foods known to contribute to the production of cancer-causing nitrosoproline (NPRO) inhibited the production of nitrosoproline. Volunteers consumed green tea along with sodium nitrate and proline, two agents that contribute to NPRO formation. Subsequent urine samples showed that the green tea consumption greatly reduced production of NPRO in the body.

Green tea also appears to protect the body from potentially damaging rays of the sun. In tests conducted at Rutgers University, green tea polyphenols inhibited the production of skin lesions caused by exposure to UVB (ultraviolet light B) rays. The same studies showed that green tea polyphenols inhibited the development of tumors caused by excessive exposure to UVB rays.

There's more. Green tea demonstrates antibacterial activity against the microbes that cause dental plaque. The polyphenols in green tea have been shown to inhibit several strains of food-borne pathogenic bacteria. This suggests that green tea may help to prevent some cases of bacterial food poisoning. Additionally, green tea promotes the growth of beneficial bifidobacteria in the intestines.

I must admit, however, that as we cruised around the emerald hills of Coonoor and walked seemingly endless tea rows, I thought little of the health benefits of tea, green or otherwise. Instead I feasted on the majesty of the plantations, with their thousands of glistening bushes, which rose up the steep sides of the ancient Nilgiri Hills in resplendent green waves.

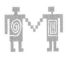

After the Nilgiris we headed south, back down into the sweltering plains, through the city of Coimbatore, into tropical Kerala state, with its millions of coconut palms, glistening green paddies, white oxen in the fields, vast plantations of cane, old stone Siva temples, goddess temples, and balmy, sweet-warm nights. Kerala is where Ayurveda began, so we were at the roots of the oldest-known system of medicine on Earth. I planned to explore some of the key Ayurvedic centers in the area.

Both Prasad and Prakash liked to eat "Andhra style," a particular manner of eating common to the southeastern Indian state of Andhra Pradesh. So on the road we looked for signs promising Andhra meals. We would enter these small restaurants, where heavy banana leaves were set on the table in front of each of us like place settings. A server would heap a large pile of rice onto the banana leaves, after which two or three different kinds of curry or lentil dahl would be poured or ladled onto the rice. Following that, several small stainless steel bowls containing additional vegetable dishes would be set down. There would also be roti, which is freshly made flat breads of buttery whole wheat, and raita, an herbed yogurt. We would eat all of this with our hands. At the end of each meal, handwashing was a necessity. We usually washed the food down with fresh lime sodas. It was an inexpensive, nutritious way to eat.

One night we stayed outside of Kottayam in a secluded garden retreat on the intercoastal waters, a vast network of lakes, canals, lagoons, and rivers that runs from the Arabian sea far inland. There men sell prawns and fish and vegetables from long, handcarved wooden boats. Traveling Indians and foreigners idle in kettuvallams, exquisite wooden houseboats with tight, finely woven bamboo roofs, windows, and doors.

A couple of days later we passed through Trivandrum—the noisy capital city of Kerala, built over seven hills—on our way south to Surya Samudra, a small resort set on a hill above the Arabian Sea. There a traditional Keralan bungalow would be our base for a week. As we rolled through lush greenery on the road to Surya Samudra, we passed hundreds of signs for beachside Ayurvedic spas offering vegetarian food, herbal cures, panchakarma massage, consultations, and treatments of different kinds. No question, the Ayurvedic boom was in full force in tropical Kerala. There by the Arabian sea, the Ayurvedic renaissance is the hippest, healthiest, happiest, most happening phenomenon in the land. Buildings of all shapes and sizes used great bold signs to advertise massages and cures. Kaboom.

At Surya Samudra we parted company with our invaluable secretary and translator, Prakash, and shaggy Prasad, our now somewhat calmer driver. "He does not drink anymore, Mr. Chris," Prakash informed me, pointing to Prasad. "Now no smoking and no drinking, in just a couple of weeks. You see what some very straight talking can do?" Prasad shyly expressed that he was happier about himself now, and that he even intended to go see a doctor about some kidney pain he was experiencing. After hugs and handshakes and rupees all around, we said goodbye to the intrepid duo.

ANCIENT METHODS, TRADITIONAL REMEDIES

Once settled into our bungalow, Shahannah and I were visited by an erudite and charming Brahman named Ramakrishna, who would help us for the next week, thanks to introductions made for us by our stateside friend Ehud Sperling, publisher of Inner Traditions books. In our first conversation, Ramakrishna proved complex, diverse, entertaining, moody, audacious, and fun. A former journalist with the *Times of India* and a producer of numerous TV documentaries, Ramakrishna is a born raconteur whose greatest pleasure is entertaining, teaching, and confounding others. He'd even done a stint as an ascetic holy man in the Himalayas "with all the devotees and ceremony that such a life entails," he noted.

"As a Brahman, do you know that I enjoy absolute privilege in Indian society?" he asked. "I can go anywhere I like, completely unchallenged. If I am away from home and need to use the toilet, I simply march up to a total stranger's door and knock. When they answer, I announce 'toilet,' with no further explanation required, and march right in and help myself. They recognize me instantaneously as a Brahman, and they simply stand aside." Whether Ramakrishna's Brahmanic heritage or his entirely bombastic manner of self-presentation was responsible, he seemed like a man who could finesse his way into almost any place.

We couldn't have found a better companion and ally. Ramakrishna helped us to set up appointments and to navigate through the systemic obfuscation and delays that typify Indian business and organizations. Over the course of a week, we traveled with Ramakrishna the raconteur, stopping at clinics, Ayurvedic massage centers, pharmacies, and herbal manufacturers, and meeting with experts of various kinds. On a couple of occasions we were met with the same irksome refusal to let us photograph that we had encountered in Bangalore. But Ramakrishna, with his silver tongue, was able to massage a few stubborn bureaucrats off the dime, and we got our shots.

Nowhere in the Trivandrum area is the traditional preparation of Ayurvedic herbal remedies as alive and thriving as at Dhanwantari Matam, an institute whose name means the abode of Dhanwantari, the patron god of Ayurveda. "You will find this place quite authentic," Ramakrishna told us. "They do things exactly according to the old scriptures, right down to the slightest details." For more than 75 years, Dhanwantari Matam has been a maker of botanical preparations, produced in accordance with traditional specifications and in small batches. The institute was founded by Sri Aranmula Narayana Pillai, a physician to the royal family of Travancore—the former native state that is now Kerala. It enjoys a distinguished reputation, and its remedies are used by top Ayurvedic practitioners throughout India.

Mr. C.P. Nair, general manager of Dhanwantari Matam, described for us the philosophy of the institute. "Ayurveda is based upon very sound principles of harmony and balance, taking into account each person's constitution and habits," he said. "As forces and conditions within the body fluctuate and change, we need those agents that can maintain and restore harmony and balance. The remedies we make contain natural ingredients because human beings respond best to products of nature. Also, we take great care to prepare our medicines according to the exact methods prescribed in the old texts, because these methods ensure quality and potency. Modern science is proving that these ancient drugs are far safer and more potent than single-molecule synthetic drugs, or drugs made from isolated plant compounds. There are no side effects with these traditional remedies."

Mr. Nair laid out upon his desk several exquisitely crafted palmyrah leaf texts, hundreds of years old, which detail the ingredients and methods of preparation for numerous traditional Ayurvedic medicines. The manuscripts were made in the most painstaking manner possible, with a sharp blade carefully used to carve small, intricate characters into the palmyrah leaves, without puncturing them. Once the tiny, detailed letters were carved, the grooves of the lettering were filled in with ink

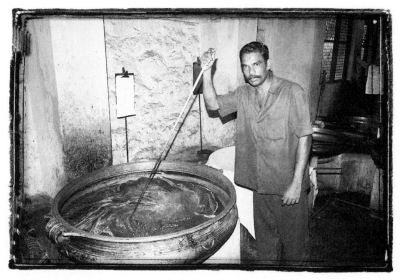

Making chyawanprash, a popular Ayurvedic remedy

applied from a single, carefully inked hair. Years were required to complete one perfect manuscript. "It used to be that every 300 years or so, these manuscripts would be remade," Mr. Nair told us. "But there is nobody to undertake this kind of work anymore. These are the last." He then invited us to see for ourselves how Dhanwantari Matam produced medicines by traditional methods.

The flow of manufacture begins with the herbs themselves. Brought in from growers and suppliers primarily from south India, herbs are cleaned, dried when necessary, sorted, sifted, chopped, and made ready for further processing. From there, the herbs are blended into powdered formulas, boiled liquid preparations, alcohol-based elixirs, oil-based remedies, or pastes.

One such paste is the famous chyawanprash, a mainstay of Ayurveda used as an all-around invigorating, preventive, health-building daily tonic. The formula, which comes in a gooey paste

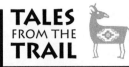

Chyawanprash

Chyawanprash, a mix of plants that comes in a gooey, vitality-enhancing paste, is to Ayurveda what peanut butter is to a well-stocked kitchen. I've seen a jar of chyawanprash in every Indian home I've been in. It can be in yours, too. You can find chyawanprash in the United States, mostly in Indian specialty stores. I take the Dabur brand myself. There are others, but I cannot vouch for them one way or the other.

Chyawanprash has a sweet, tangy flavor that is delicious. Because chyawanprash spreads easily, you can spread it on toast (my favorite) or crackers. Or you can just eat a spoonful once or twice daily.

with a pleasant, tangy flavor, is a staple health-enhancer used ubiquitously throughout India. Dabur brand chyawanprash, one of India's most popular brands, promises to "strengthen you from deep within." The unique flavor of chyawanprash comes from its base of amla, a tart, cherry-size fruit that is unusually rich in vitamin C. In addition to amla, chyawanprash usually contains a couple dozen herbs—including ashwagandha, of course.

Many hundreds of companies make chyawanprash, but not all of them adhere to traditional recipes for the rejuvenating paste. "Here we use only fresh, ripe amla," explained one herbal blending expert at Dhanwantari Matam. "Many places will use dried amla, which is no good, or even some other fruit and sugar. We would never do that. We make the pure, traditional chyawanprash. This is why people feel good when they take our formula."

Shahannah and I were especially impressed by the slow cooking of herbs in wide, shallow brass pots, the size and shape of which are specified in Ayurvedic scriptures. Tradition dictates not only the form of these vessels but also the types of wood used for the cooking fires. This combination, typically accompanied by regular stirring and a precise cooking time, ensures just the right pace of evaporation and the right consistency and potency of finished products.

In the manufacturing area, we observed hand-filling of containers of chyawanprash and saw numerous other remedies ready for use. Dhanwantari Matam also offers consultation to patients undergoing Ayurvedic treatment, and the institute provides apprenticeships for graduates of Ayurvedic colleges who require supervision as they train in the art of consulting with patients. Mr. Nair summed up the work at Dhanwantari this way: "The tradition of Ayurveda must be kept alive. Ayurveda has thousands of years of success, so we do not have to wait for science to tell us that it works. Do you see? This is the science of life. It is already well-formed. We are carrying that tradition in today's modern world. We are making medicines that heal. This is our sacred mission."

When we weren't running around to Ayurvedic places large and small with Ramakrishna, Shahannah and I took a little time to relax by the azure Arabian Sea, watching fishermen in small log boats setting nets on the undulating swells. In the mornings, crows would make sudden runs at our coffee cups as we sat on a tile veranda overlooking the water. Twice they made off with the sugar bowl. In the evenings, musicians came to

Surya Samudra to play traditional classical music. We would sit with a warm breeze blowing, listening to the sounds of crashing waves as sweet music from bamboo flutes floated gracefully in the evening air.

At Surya Samudra we also saw traditional kattakali dancers, men who represent gods and goddesses in scenes from Hindu religious epics like the Mahabarata and Ramayana. Women do not perform in these religious dramas. The kattakali dancers wear elaborate makeup that takes hours to make and apply. All afternoon we watched the men pulverize brightly colored roots and stones with pestles and mortars, making fine powders that would be mixed with water or oil and then applied to the face in elaborate fashion. After spending hours on the makeup, the men donned huge, cumbersome costumes of robes, ballooned undergirding, leggings, and huge headgear. They looked like beings from a cosmic dreamworld. Kattakali dances are the soap operas of the gods. On a stone platform overlooking the sea, the actors performed scenes from an epic, employing stylized dance while a priest chanted narration and drummers beat rhythm and clanged cymbals. It was truly wonderful.

A STROLL THROUGH THE BOTANICAL GARDEN

Outside Trivandrum, in the town of Palode, we journeyed with Ramakrishna to a spectacular botanical garden established for the preservation and investigation of the flora of south India. The Tropical Botanical Garden and Research Institute (TBGRI) is home to a world-class collection of tropical plants, and it's a center of busy research into the medicinal applications of many south Indian species. Shahannah and I had heard about TBGRI through a much-publicized project conducted by a Dr. Rajasekharan, head of the institute's ethnomedicine division. The project, which resulted in the marketing of a formula called Jeevani, was the first in India in which a percentage of sales went to natives from whose tradition the central herbal ingredient originated. In an area surrounded by verdant hills, singing birds, and the fragrances of flower blossoms, TBGRI sat like a lustrous jewel in the crown of the region.

Dr. Rajasekharan greeted us warmly, and after the ubiquitous and much-welcome cup of tea, he shared with us the story of his collaboration with the Kani people, a hill tribe whose medicinal plant knowledge led to the development of Jeevani. "Two of us from the Tropical Botanical Garden were hiking in the Agastya Hills with a couple of members of the Kani tribe back in 1987," he related. "The conditions were a bit difficult, with steep climbing. We were finding it very difficult to keep going, but the tribespeople did not seem even the slightest bit fatigued. We asked them how they kept their energy going, and they showed us some small green berries. We had seen our guides chewing these along the way. I chewed a small handful, and right then I felt a sudden flush of energy and strength."

Dr. Rajasekharan knew that the plant had real sales potential if it proved to be safe. The berries came from *Tricopus zeylanicus*, a plant the Kani call aarogyappacha. The TBGRI researched the plant, which, as far as could be determined, grows only in the hills of Kerala. Working with a company called Arya Veda Pharmacy, the researchers devised a tonic formula called Jeevani, which means source of life. "It took us 8 years to research and develop a product that we knew was safe and effective for promoting energy and relieving fatigue," explained Dr. Rajasekharan. Jeevani contains ashwagandha, black pepper, a couple of other herbs, and *Tricopus zeylanicus*, the green, energy-imbuing berry of the Kani tribe. The product comes in granules. You take half a teaspoon of it and mix it in hot water or hot milk and drink it down.

In accordance with a 1992 United Nations Convention on Biological Diversity, TBGRI decided to share profits from the Jeevani product with the Kani tribespeople. "We knew that we were doing the right thing," says TBGRI's director, P. Pushpangadan. Doing the right thing so flew in the face of common practice that the project made international news. In most cases, native people around the world are completely exploited for their medicinal plant knowledge, typically receiving little or nothing in return. For the Kani, payday has already come, if modestly. The Kani received their first payment of $12,500 in 1999, with further proceeds to follow on an annual basis.

On a tour of the large medicinal plant section of the botanical garden, Dr. Rajasekharan proudly showed us several displays of plants grouped together. Anti-inflammatory plants were growing in one garden, ingredients for chyawanprash, the popular herbal paste, were clustered in another, while anti-diabetic herbs occupied yet another growing area.

We saw about 100 different Ayurvedic plants, including ashwagandha, aloe vera, gotu kola (*Centella asiatica*), cinnamon, and black pepper. And we saw *Bacopa monnieri*, which we had not previously encountered. In the state of Kerala, where *Bacopa* grows, it is known as brahmi, a tonic herb reputed to improve intelligence and memory and revitalize the sense organs. *Bacopa*, or brahmi, is also credited with restoring youthful vitality and improving digestion. Like ashwagandha, it is a tonic used to improve overall health, energy, stamina, sex, and brain function. A creeping, herbaceous plant common in marshes and backwaters, *Bacopa* contains the alkaloids brahmine and herpestine, plus a group of novel compounds known as bacosides A and B, monnierin, and bacogenin A1, A2, and A3. Researchers at TBGRI seemed especially interested in its possible value in reducing age-related degeneration of the eyes. Its traditional use in Ayurveda for eye disease has led to further inquiry into the use of *Bacopa* to help maintain eye health and good vision into old age. With such a long history of benefit to the brain and eyes, the plant may become one of the most popular botanicals in the Ayurvedic category.

In the garden, signs stressed the importance of medicinal plant preservation, the cultivation of medicinal plants, different traditional uses of certain plants, or their unusual properties. "Our purpose here is to make sure that these valuable plants remain available, and that research into their medicinal uses continues," Dr. Rajasekharan explained. "We are dedicated to this work. We hope to initiate more work like the Jeevani project, in time developing other medicines. There are so many valuable plants that can help people with common health problems."

As we strolled the beautiful gardens and took pictures, I got the sense that TBGRI enjoyed some sort of divine protection, and that the center would continue to be a fountain of good botanical works. As if to emphasize the point, a beautiful black statue of Dhanwantari, the patron god of Ayurveda, stands on a hilltop overlooking the medicinal plant gardens.

During a brief respite after our trip to TBGRI, Shahannah and I spent some time at Kovalam beach, a mecca for economy tourists, hippies, inveterate road gypsies, and nomadic global citizens. Smaller than Goa and less traveled, Kovalam is a thriving center of hip Ayurvedic culture. There, along the beach, Ayurveda has become as popular as rock and roll and as faddish as disco in the 1970s. Every hotel, motel, guest house, and bungalow along this popular resting spot offered herb-infused Ayurvedic massages, consultations, vegetarian food, and complete rejuvenation packages. One building in particular stands out in my mind. The Arya Ayurvedic Center, made of rough red brick and covered by a palm-leaf roof, advertised oil massage, yoga, and panchakarma treatment. Running along the front of the entire place was a brightly painted red wall that proclaimed "Real Refresher! Coca-Cola." We didn't need the confirmation, but this was a clear sign that in funky Kovalam by the Arabian Sea, Ayurveda is the real thing.

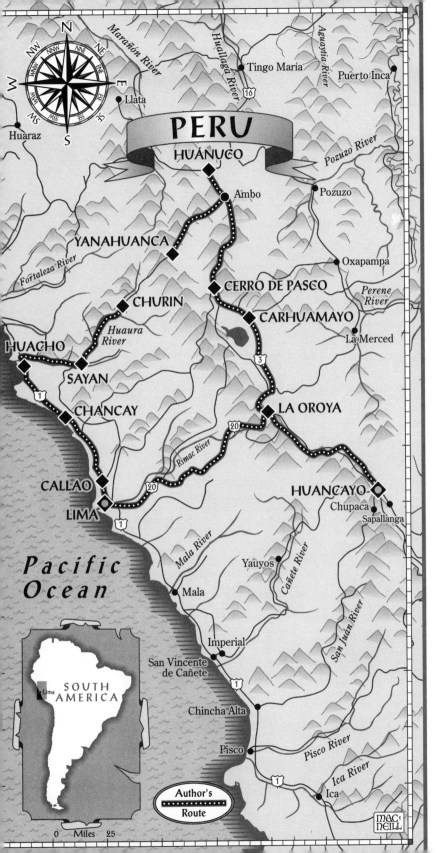

On the Maca Trail

THE ROAD TO CHURIN

The South American country of Peru, with its extraordinarily diverse terrain, is one of the richest nations in the world in plant life. Peru weighs in with 1,500 miles of desert coastline, a vast Amazon rain forest, mountains as high as 22,000 feet, and the world's highest navigable lake, Lake Titicaca.

The varying climates and altitudes of Peru yield a high volume of agricultural crops, from cane to asparagus to jasmine. Peru's tradition of medicinal plant use is also rich. In the jungles and Amazon River basin within Peru, shamans and native plant experts employ hundreds of botanicals for medicinal and nutritional purposes. And in one of the most inhospitable environments of Peru, the Central Highlands, a legendary plant passed down from the Incas is about to become a major botanical success story and popular product. That plant is maca.

My wife Shahannah and I were in Peru on behalf of Pure-World Botanicals to explore the maca trail. Although it's often dubbed Peruvian ginseng, maca bears no botanical relation to ginseng. But, like ginseng, maca is reputed to increase strength, energy, stamina, libido, and sexual function—a winning combination of health benefits if there ever was one. Still, low crop yields or onerous logistical difficulties can keep even a very healthful plant from being a marketable product. From what I already knew, I suspected that maca had a bright future as a dietary supplement in the huge U.S. market, but our investigations would help us to know this for certain.

From Boston, 10 hours of flying put us into Lima, Peru's capital, late at night. We collected our luggage and were met by Sergio Cam and his wife Techi. Sergio could easily be mistaken for a Navajo, with his classic native face and shoulder-length black hair. For several years, Sergio worked in the United States for 6 months out of the year, building houses north of San Francisco. He speaks Spanish, English, and some Quechua, the major indigenous language of the region. His involvement with maca started when a shaman gave him some of the plant in the Peruvian town of Nazca. "He told me that the maca would change things for me, and it did," Sergio recalled. Taking up the maca trade as his calling, Sergio left his lucrative contracting work and now works full-time with maca growers in the Peruvian highlands. These days, Sergio Cam is *the* maca connection.

At the airport, the four of us crowded into a red Toyota Hilux four-wheel-drive pickup truck and set off through miles of dismal gray industrial miasma with deserted streets, high concrete walls, and ominous fencing topped with double layers of barbed and razor wires. "This area is dangerous," remarked Sergio. I believed him.

Once into the heart of Lima, we trucked down broad avenues with wrought-iron lamp posts in the misty night. Our hotel—the Gran Bolivar—sat at one end of the Plaza San Martin like a great spotlit colonial monarch. Inside, past the foyer, a majestic marble hall crowned by a spectacular stained-glass ro-

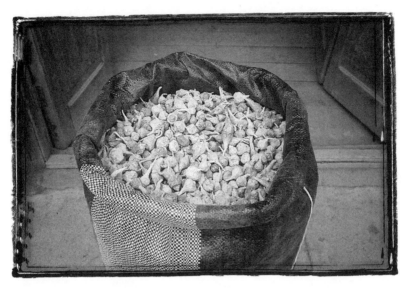
Maca drying in a storage bag

tunda, all under renovation, spoke of a previous time when the hotel was the crown jewel of Lima, a South American must-stop for celebrities, statesmen, diplomats, and other luminaries.

We followed a cheerful red-capped bellman pushing a luggage cart along mahogany-trimmed hallways to an inexpensive fourth-floor suite. Shahannah and I were the only guests on the entire cavernous floor. There was a large sitting room and an impressive-looking bathroom with a deep tub. The whole place smelled of mildew and dust, so we flung the windows open wide and took in Lima's caustic, polluted air through thin, old drapes. Shahannah and I fell fast into deep sleep, oblivious to the noisy night of sirens, yells, shots, and tire screeches.

INTO THE HILLS

In the morning, a friend of Sergio's named Rubén picked us up in the red Toyota truck. Rubén tied our luggage into the bed and then climbed in back to keep it safe. We sped over to Sergio's house, where we saw Techi and their two small daughters, Masha and Amy. Techi, with long sandy-blond hair, a beaming smile, and a friendly, easy-going manner, is quick to laugh and a pleasure to be around. Sometimes she travels with Sergio, but more often she stays in Lima with their children.

There we also met a shaman friend of Sergio's named Enrique. Sergio had decided that we would travel with him, Techi, and Enrique to the hot springs at Churin, where we could relax, unwind, and rejuvenate ourselves in natural bubbling springs. "You're going to like this place a lot," Sergio proclaimed. "These hot springs at Churin are famous. They are where Fujimori, the president of Peru, goes. The ride is a little long, but it's not too bad and the scenery is nice."

The five of us tied our luggage into the back of the Toyota, squeezed ourselves into the king cab, and headed off to Churin.

Traffic ran heavy and fast, with cars, trucks, buses, and bicycle carts jammed at intersections. Thousands of banana-yellow taxicabs hustled and blared. Old American Chevys, Fords, and Dodges—with wired-on bumpers, dragging tailpipes, and roaring, punctured mufflers—belched black exhaust as they rattled and heaved. Some buses appeared like ghost vehicles from another period in history, hulking metal heaps from the 1940s with rusted roofs and bald tires. Many trucks were well over 50 years old, rumbling along with huge, high loads that swayed from side to side, often with 10 to 20 people riding on top—not to mention luggage, furniture, produce, chickens, bicycles, and all manner of goods. At intersections drivers leaned on their horns for minutes at a time, for no apparent reason. The honking, the hee-haw and weepu-weepu of sirens, and the sputter and roar of engines of all sizes combined like ill-tuned instruments in a drunken orchestra.

The abundance of armed, uniformed men in the city was unsettling. Almost all police wore bullet-proof vests, and many sported evil-looking high-tech automatic rifles. All along the boulevards there were police cars, large police trucks, caged police wagons, and slate-gray riot tanks with heavy armor and slit windows.

As we approached the edge of town, we purchased petrol and bottled water. We then drove north, up the barren, sandy coast along Peru Route 1. We passed through the cities of Callao and Chancay and remained northbound until we reached Huacho, a large city not too far up the coast from Lima where fishing vessels operate. From Huacho we turned inland toward Sayan, along the Huaura River.

Now heading east into a countryside rich with arable land, we passed small and large fields of soccer ball–size cauliflower, great green cabbage, lettuce, and broccoli. We admired huge fields of asparagus, multi-hectare plots of scallions, and vast acreage of green peppers, chilies, and tomatoes. Corn fields and cane fields stretched for miles, interrupted by stands of fennel, potato fields, and plots of leafy greens. Brilliant fields of marigolds provided a rich shock of orange. We motored past acres of beautiful yellow roses as well as several jasmine orchards, whose exotic, sweet perfume wafted through the air. Small boys tended large herds of goats, and we saw sheep, small groups of cattle, and donkeys. Field-workers toiled with hand tools, hoes, shovels, rakes, and clippers, packing crops into crates, boxes, and bags.

The soil in the Peruvian countryside is terrifically rocky; there are rock walls and piles everywhere. But the soil is fertile enough to yield abundant crops, and the people are skilled farmers who know how to grow food. Still, an increasing number of stores sell fertilizers, pesticides, and fungicides, which pollute soil and water, endanger the health of farm workers, and kill wildlife. The chemical companies are crafty marketers, and they are discovering in Peru a growth market for their hazardous and often counterproductive soil adjuncts and chemical inputs.

The journey to Churin requires a minimum of 6 hours in the best of circumstances, and it put us on a long, lonely road that was among the very worst I have ever traveled. Rutted, uneven, intensely dusty, strewn with rocks, and too narrow in most spots for two-way traffic, the road frequently washed out, relocated, dropped off hillsides into river beds, and fell apart. Large mining trucks bore down on us from ahead and behind, and passing was often extremely hairy.

Steep earth and rock hillsides towering beside the roads bore evidence of slides, which can bury or crush a vehicle under hundreds of tons of stone. In a couple of places, the road became a slope of scree that slid down into the bed of the Huaura River. We had to stop a few times along the way just to stand and stretch and give our kidneys a rest from constant jarring.

As we pressed on, the road deteriorated into a torture track. The Toyota bounced, banged, and skidded along, throwing up churning spumes of dust. Eventually the road washed out altogether, gone in a huge slide of mud and rocks, erased by the shifting of a whole mountainside. As we rode along the dry bed of the river, dust painted us a muddy brown, like theater makeup for the role of unwashed bums.

Sayan, a crossroads town of numerous fruit stands, roadside restaurants, and dogs, has a couple of places where a blown tire can be repaired. Since seemingly half the vehicles on Peru's roads are careening along on bald tires, the tire repair business is a boom industry. Somehow, though, we overshot Sayan and had to backtrack to it for a quick lunch of turkey, rice, beans, and slivered onions before resuming our campaign to Churin. Periodically we'd stop to ask how far away Churin was. The answers varied from 2 hours to half an hour to 20 minutes to 5 hours.

The anticipation of a soothing hot mineral bath made our assault on the highlands more bearable. Around 7:30 in the evening, we hauled up a steep gravel grade across which arched a sign welcoming us to Churin, thus ending our 8-hour drive. Without ado, we headed straight to the only hot spring still open, in the lightless basement of an old concrete building that reeked of urine and mildew. Before descending, we entered a changing area, where Shahannah tugged on my shirt. "What's that over there?" she asked with horror. I looked closely. More than one person had crapped on the floor in the corner of the locker room. We opted to change elsewhere.

Techi passed on the bath. The rest of us were not as wise, and we descended a slippery set of stairs into the basement gloom. I stood directly in front of a hole in the wall through which spring water flowed into the basement. There our dusty little group soaked off road dirt with little cheer in tepid, foul-smelling waters, while an irritated attendant in rubber boots stood at the top of the stairs shaking a broom angrily and telling us we should get out of there so he could go home. I burst out laughing at the whole pathetic scene and wondered, as I do at moments when I find myself way out in the middle of nowhere in some marginal situation, just what the heck I was doing here.

After our lukewarm hot spring experience, we walked into the center of tiny, rural Churin for *chifa*—Chinese food. The restaurant was located next door to our little hotel, Las Termas. You can find decent Chinese food even in many of the smallest villages in Peru; the Chinese who worked on the Peruvian railways in the 1800s brought their cuisine with them.

Over dinner, we learned a little bit about Enrique. Slightly taller than Sergio, Enrique is a bit stocky and has a head of thick, ink-black hair. His relaxed face and alert eyes give him the appearance of being simultaneously friendly and watchful. Enrique works as a computer programmer at a hospital in Lima to support his family, but his psychic intuition and healing skills—and his ability to travel back and forth between the material and spirit worlds—make him a sought-after shaman.

Describing to us the event that changed the course of his life, Enrique told us, "At age 7, I was climbing up a hill in the highlands when I was struck unconscious by a bolt of lightning. One moment I was walking, and the next moment I was knocked down, just like that. When I came to, I was in the care of two shamans who regarded the lightning strike as an auspicious sign that I was meant to tread the path of traditional spiritual wisdom. Those two men taught me for many years." Enrique's hand gestures are extravagantly expressive, and he frequently swirls his arm overhead as if to sculpt a spiral in the air when speaking about spiritual insight and energy. "I see from the third eye, the pineal gland," he said, pressing the pad of his index finger into the center of his forehead. "From here I can see into the spiritual realms."

After this discussion, Shahannah and I retired to Las Termas, where we huddled against the mountain cold in a tiny but clean single bed. I awoke in the morning with a row of itchy red bug bites along my left arm, which terminated in a puffy, egg-size lump. "What is that?" Shahannah asked. "Cooties," I replied.

Shortly past 6:00 our little group ambled up the town's narrow main road to a small restaurant for coffee. We were served cups of hot water, and Shahannah and I looked around expectantly for the coffee. "That's the coffee there," Sergio helped out, pointing to a small glass vessel resembling a soy sauce dispenser, filled with dark liquid. The idea was to pour a little bit of the liquid, which turned out to be regular-strength coffee, into the hot water. The resulting cup looked like tannic stream water, with a weak aroma, little taste, and no jolt.

If the previous evening's soak in stale waters was unsatisfying, our morning journey to an attractive and clean hot spring spa by a small river made up for the experience in spades. Doors on individual rooms displayed signs that read hot, hotter, and very hot, prompting Sergio to predict with a laugh, "I think this place is going to be a lot better than the one last night." Shahannah and I chose a "hotter" room. The water had a pleasant sulfuric aroma, but it was so scalding that I could only marvel at the notion that anyone would actually try to get into it. Only after we tempered the scalding water with tens of gallons of frigid spring water were we able to even get into the 5-foot-square sunken tile tub to soak our cares—and almost our lobster-red skin—away.

Toweled off and rag-doll relaxed, we had fortune smile upon us with our very first maca experience. At a small bar at the spa, a woman was making blender drinks that consisted of cooked maca, honey, vanilla extract, and a little quinoa, a nutritious Peruvian grain. The drink was delicious, with a viscous consistency and a mildly sweet, nutty flavor. I was so enamored with it that I downed the first tall glass of it and had another. Maybe it was my imagination, but I swear that the drink made me feel vigorous and full of energy. I walked outside and did stretching exercises, working the kinks out of my body. I felt magnificent.

As it turns out, blender drinks are among the most common ways that maca is consumed in Peru. Only urban dwellers resort to capsules of maca powder. Most Peruvians who benefit from the plant consume it as a food. You can walk into any town and find at least one place selling maca blender drinks.

Maca, *Lepidium meyenii*, is the only cruciferous plant native to Peru. The cruciferous plants include rapeseed (the source of canola oil), radish, cauliflower, cabbage, Brussels sprouts, watercress, and a number of other important food crops. Maca is an annual plant that produces a radishlike tuber that matures within approximately 7 months after seeds are planted. Maca root has a sweet, nutty flavor and is typically dried and stored. It will easily keep for 7 years. The dried, ground-up form of maca is usually used in Peru—as a breakfast cereal, in baked goods, in blender drinks, and even in alcoholic beverages.

Little is known about the origins of maca, but the plant is believed to have been cultivated in the Junin Plateau of the Central Highlands in pre-Incan times, as far back as 2,000 years ago. The Spanish conquest of Peru that began in 1526 included a campaign of cultural destruction, which ultimately resulted in the demise of the Incan empire. The Inca were sophisticated architects, builders, and cultivators of the land. They had established a highly developed society that worshiped the sun, and their prodigious works, seen in the ruins at Machu Picchu, remain among the wonders of the world to this day. Among the many treasures held by the Incas and garnered by the Spanish was maca. The Inca considered maca to be a gift from the gods. They so prized the plant that it was used as a form of currency.

When Spanish conquistadores ventured into Peru's Central Highlands, they became concerned for the health and fertility of their livestock, especially the horses. In those high altitudes there were no grasslands for grazing, and the thin air and hostile climate produced a precipitous drop in animal fertility. The Incas recommended that the Spanish feed their horses maca. The Spanish followed this advice and were thus able to keep their horses well-nourished and to return their fertility back to normal. The Spanish were deeply impressed.

Also to their surprise, the Spanish found strong, healthy babies and adults in the hostile highlands, a condition attributable to a diet consisting mostly of maca, which is a balanced food rich in carbohydrates, protein, and fatty acids. The Incas, and subsequently the Spanish, used maca as a staple food and fed it to livestock. The

The famous Incan ruins at Machu Picchu

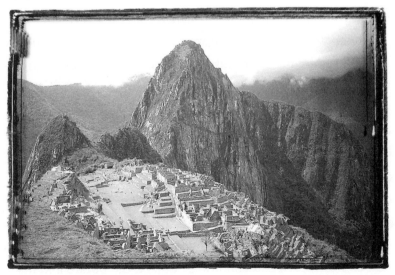

Spanish didn't take long to figure out that whatever was in maca that enhanced animal fertility might likely promote a sexual effect in humans. In maca they discovered a worthy aphrodisiac.

Legend has it that during the height of the Incan empire, warriors would consume maca before entering into battle. This would make them fiercely strong. But after conquering a city, the Incan soldiers were prohibited from using maca. That was to protect the conquered women. So from at least as far back as 500 years ago, maca's reputation for enhancing strength, libido, and fertility was already well-established in Peru.

Today, maca's popularity is spreading to the general population of Peru—native and non-native alike. And market demand is being created in Japan, Europe, and the United States. As a result, maca cultivation is on the increase, with a number of Peruvian government experts and agencies promoting maca agriculture and development. Clearly, maca is poised to be a major botanical product on the international herbal scene.

Maca grows in a limited geographic area at elevations between 10,000 and 15,000 feet, such as the Junin Plateau, where approximately 1,000 acres of maca are grown annually, mostly in small family plots. Because of the growing demand, agricultural experts predict that the acreage dedicated to maca cultivation will steadily increase to 123,500 acres early in this century. The Junin Plateau, however, is notorious for its hostile conditions. Temperatures often plunge below zero, large hailstones and slushy snow commonly fall in the summer, the oxygen-thin air induces altitude sickness, the rocky soil supports very little plant life, the wind chaps the skin, and the glaring sun can burn you red in minutes. But maca is unusually frost-resistant and thrives in bad conditions. In fact, the potato and maca

Maca, the Libido Lifter

What's in maca that promotes its sex-enhancing effects? Science hasn't solved the mystery for sure, but there are some candidates.

Isothiocyanates are found in the root of maca as well as in other cruciferous plants such as horseradish, mustard, and radishes. These compounds induce protective phase 2 enzymes, which fight cancer by detoxifying carcinogens and eliminating them from the body. Maca contains benzyl thiocyanate and p-methoxybenzyl isothiocyanate in small amounts, which may also enhance fertility.

Alkaloids have been mentioned as possibly playing a role in maca's sex-enhancing effects. This notion originates from the 1961 publication of a paper by maca researcher Gloria Chacon de Popavici, who claims to have found certain alkaloids in maca. But recent in-depth chemical investigation into maca employing state-of-the-art technology reveals no such alkaloids. If maca does contain alkaloids, they occur in undetectably minute amounts.

Macamides and *macaenes* are the names given to two groups of novel compounds in maca discovered by a team of analytical chemists at PureWorld Botanicals. Preliminary experiments with animals point to these compounds as likely sex and energy enhancers. In the experiments, sexual activity and stamina increased significantly as the quantities of macamides and macaenes in the diet increased.

---

are the only crops that grow in the Junin Plateau's altitude range. My more intense field work on maca would begin with a trip up to Junin—after our little vacation in Churin was over.

The most referred-to paper on maca originated from Naples, Italy, and was published in *Food Chemistry* in 1994. The paper, entitled "Chemical Composition of *Lepidium meyenii*," describes the rich nutritional value of maca and makes sense of how the Peruvians in the Central Highlands can subsist on this

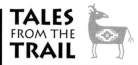

How Much Maca Should You Take? A Lot!

In the United States, you can find maca in powdered form, tablets, capsules, and liquids. But when you take maca as a supplement, does it work the way it works for Peruvians who eat it as food? It's mostly a matter of dosage.

Peruvians who eat maca as porridge, chew on maca tubers, or consume blended maca drinks typically get 5 grams to perhaps 2 ounces or more per serving. But supplement companies put only about 500 milligrams of ground, dried maca in each capsule and recommend three to six capsules daily. Rare is the herb that works in such small doses. I believe that to get any benefit from maca, you'd need to take a minimum of 5 grams—10 capsules of 500 milligrams each—of powdered maca daily.

With MacaPure, a standardized, concentrated extract of maca, you can take less because it contains a specific concentration of macamides and macaenes, the novel compounds in maca that have been shown to enhance sexual activity in tests with animals. Companies selling MacaPure are recommending two 450-milligram capsules of MacaPure extract daily. I'd say that's the absolute minimum to take, and I would recommend double that amount, or around 2 grams daily. (For information on where to buy MacaPure and other maca products, see Resources on page 281.)

In toxicity studies conducted in the United States, maca showed absolutely no toxicity and no adverse pharmacologic effects. So you can be generous with the amounts of maca products you take—I definitely am.

tuber. Dried maca weighs in at about 59 percent carbohydrate and has a protein value of slightly more than 10 percent. It possesses a higher content of beneficial fatty acids—primarily linoleic acid, palmitic acid, and oleic acid—than other root crops. Maca is also a rich source of healthful sterols, including sitosterol, campestrol, ergosterol, brassicasterol, and ergostadienol. From a mineral standpoint, maca exceeds both potatoes and carrots in value, and it is a good source of iron, magnesium, calcium, potassium, and iodine.

According to folklore, maca is just about a panacea. Peruvians claim that maca stimulates metabolism (perhaps as a result of its thyroid-stimulating iodine), regulates hormonal secretion (possibly the work of isothyacyanates and sterols), improves memory (maybe owing to certain amino acids), combats anemia (most likely because of its high iron value), and fights depression (perhaps because of its amino acids and minerals). It's also touted as a laxative (probably from its fiber content) and as a cure for rheumatism and respiratory disorders. And, of course, maca is sold as an aphrodisiac and to boost strength, promote stamina, and enhance fertility.

Of all the claims made for maca, those that have been corroborated in the lab concern stamina and sexual function. In animal experiments, rodents fed maca demonstrated increased energy and exhibited an exponential increase in sexual activity as compared with animals that weren't fed maca. Though no formal studies have been conducted on maca's use for hormonal enhancement, some physicians claim success with maca for exactly this purpose.

For Sergio, developing the maca market means more than producing a cash crop. "Maca is not just a product," he told me. "It's also a spirit. Many people want maca right now, but maybe some of them don't respect the culture of the growers, or they don't care for the spiritual world. I think those people are going to have problems. But I believe that the right people will feel this spirit, and that the maca business and opportunity for the campesinos (the peasant growers) is going to work out. In the long run, I think that we will do well because we connect with those people and we want to help them to maintain their culture and their spiritual values. This is their opportunity."

Sergio's connection of maca's potential economic benefit with its spiritual value is a reflection of centuries of Peruvian tradition. The Incas thought of maca as a direct gift from the gods—and the campesinos of the highlands still do today. The reason they consider the presence of maca to be divine providence is simple—it keeps them alive. So a successful maca market would be just another way for maca to do what it always has done—provide these people with sustenance.

After our gratifying morning hot-spring soak and our first delightful experience with maca, we once again packed ourselves into the Toyota for the 8-hour drive back to Lima. On the way out of Churin, we passed a silver pickup filled with garbage and backed up to the edge of the road. A man in high rubber boots stood in the garbage, using a rake to drag the refuse out of the truck and push it down the river bank. He waved and smiled as we drove by. We waved back—and watched mounds of trash tumble into the flowing mountain water.

Our brief and restful vacation at the hot springs of Churin was over. It was time to regear for more serious maca investigation. It was time to get to work.

AT A MACA FESTIVAL

Two days after our holiday in Churin, Sergio, Shahannah, Rubén, and I jammed ourselves and our gear into the Toyota and set off east from Lima for Cerro de Pasco, the largest center of maca commerce in Peru's Central Highlands. As we climbed steadily on narrow two-lane paved roads, the air grew cooler and I noticed more vegetation on the hills. We gained even more altitude and the hillsides around us grew higher, the drops off the sides of the road fell farther down, and the switchbacks became steeper. Mining trucks and buses barreled at us around blind corners. For most of the ride, an overcast sky cast a blanket of gray over the landscape—odd weather, I thought, for October, which is spring in that part of the world.

Upward we climbed, winding our way around the mountains and traversing great grassy valleys, many of which afforded spectacular views of snowcapped Andean peaks. At hundreds of places, horsetail waterfalls cascaded down steep, rocky slopes. The Andes' yearlong runoff of melted snow, along with countless springs bubbling up through rock fissures at high elevations, creates a watery world of streams, brooks, waterfalls, vigorous rivers, and rivulets all seeking lower ground. At times, streams passed right across the road in a pell-mell downward rush.

We stopped a couple of times to stretch our compressed spines and drink coca leaf tea, the national beverage of Peru. The tea, mild in flavor and slightly green in the cup, is a rich source of valuable dietary flavonoids and phenols that protect cells, help to maintain capillary integrity, and enhance heart health. It also imparts a tiny amount of naturally occurring cocaine, which helps to allay the fatiguing effects of less oxygen at higher altitudes. The stimulating effect of coca leaf tea is actually less than plain tea, but it proved refreshing and helped us adjust to the thinner atmosphere.

Coca is sacred to the Peruvians. According to native tradition, Manco Capac, the divine son of the Sun itself, descended from his seat in the cliffs surrounding Lake Titicaca to bestow blessings upon the poor people who inhabited that land. In addition to providing the people with useful arts and the practice of agriculture, Manco Capac gave them coca to alleviate their hunger, allay their fatigue, and inspire the weary at heart.

For Peruvians, coca leaf is a godsend, and they scoff at the notion that it should be eradicated. They cultivate the coca bush, *Erythroxylum coca*, in plantations called cocals, which can be large or small. Women and children are typically employed to collect the leaves, picking them off the branches and stuffing them into cloth sacks, much like harvesting tea. As a hot infusion, coca leaf tea resembles green tea, with its pleasant aroma and mildly astringent taste. Many Peruvians use coca leaf in the form of a quid, a group of leaves placed in the cheek of the mouth along with a little lime, which helps free small amounts of the naturally occurring cocaine from the cells of the leaf. With just coca leaves and a meager amount of food, Peruvians can travel great distances on foot and perform strenuous labor with minimum fatigue.

When the Spanish first came to Peru in the 16th century, they ventured into the interior, where the native Peruvians, to whom the plant was considered a divine gift, cultivated coca with reverence and care. Priests used the leaves in virtually all ceremonies and rituals, and it was considered foolhardy to attempt to propitiate the gods without giving respect to coca by employing it in the process. The leaf was so highly valued that it was used as currency. But the Spanish mocked its cultivation by the Peruvians and in the 1560s made attempts to eradicate it in the belief that the plant and its use were inherently evil. These efforts were to little avail. Eventually, Spanish laboring in the thin atmosphere of the Peruvian highlands discovered the fatigue-allaying virtues of the plant and became its users instead of its persecutors.

In 1722, Antonio Julian, a Jesuit priest, published a book entitled *Perla de America,* in which he praised coca as a more beneficial alternative to coffee and tea. In 1793, physician Don Pedro Rolasco Crespo wrote a pamphlet praising the salutary virtues of coca and recommending it for use by sailors. Baron Ernst Von Bibra, a pioneering researcher in the field of mind-altering plants, wrote about coca in 1855, bringing the plant further to the attention of the European scientific and medical community.

Coca leaf's relation to global society changed forever when cocaine, the primary alkaloid in coca responsible for the leaf's invigorating effects, was isolated by German chemist Albert Niemann in 1860. Suddenly, a highly potent stimulant was available in concentrated form to a world that was not prepared for it. A veritable blizzard of cocaine-fortified products gained prominence in Europe and the United States. Among the most popular of these was Vin Tonique Mariani, patented in the 1860s by a chemist named Angelo Mariani from the Mediterranean island of Corsica. Ulysses S. Grant consumed Vin Tonique Mariani in milk daily near the end of his life. President William McKinley, inventor Thomas Edison, and writers Jules Verne and H.G. Wells also turned to the elixir for inspiration. Sigmund Freud, a user, wrote a popular treatise, "On Coca," in 1884.

Cocaine was Christmas morning for drug giant Parke-Davis, which took up with alacrity and dispatch the task of dispensing the drug to an eager American public. In the 1880s, Parke-Davis released a plethora of products, including candies, tablets, sprays, gargles, and ointments—all containing pure cocaine.

COCA AND THE REAL THING

The most important step toward everyday consumption by the American public of the coca leaf's stimulating alkaloid came when an unknown Atlanta pharmacist named Asa Griggs Chandler purchased a patent in 1891 for a formula that would become known as Coca-Cola. For 25 years, the Coca-Cola Company of Atlanta's best-selling soda provided the masses with a combined jolt of cocaine from coca leaf and caffeine from kola nut. Not surprisingly, Coca-Cola became popular as a stimulant par excellence. Physicians touted it as a health drink, and to this day people reach for the soda to quell an uneasy stomach and to relieve hangovers.

In 1906, with government policy moving against legal use of the drug, the Coca-Cola Company prudently removed the cocaine from its soda. In 1922, cocaine became classified in the United States as a narcotic. Though the designation was scientifically inaccurate—cocaine, a stimulant alkaloid, produces exactly the opposite effects of a drowsiness-inducing narcotic—cocaine had gone overnight from being a legal consumer product to an illicit drug.

Nearly a century after the elimination of cocaine from Coca-Cola, the Coca-Cola Company remains the sole user of coca leaf extract (minus the cocaine) in the United States. Coca-Cola owes its unique flavor to a nutritious coca leaf extract supplied to the beverage giant by the Stepan Company of Maywood, New Jersey, the nation's sole legal processor of coca leaf. Coca-Cola is unduplicated because of its proprietary use of coca-leaf extract. Without it, imitators fall short of reproducing the unique taste of "The Real Thing." In Peru, you can walk into a restaurant or approach a roadside stand and enjoy coca leaf, with its naturally occurring small amounts of invigorating cocaine, without problem. But for those in the United States who want legal access to the health-imbuing properties of coca leaf, Coca-Cola is the only game in town.

Coca leaf has been an object of controversy for centuries, and it still is. Used in its whole form, coca leaf is a fundamentally benign herbal material that provides vitamin A, riboflavin, iron, and calcium. It may also help to regulate blood glucose, thus enhancing metabolism and helping to reduce the tendency toward adult-onset diabetes and obesity. But its concentrated, isolated alkaloid cocaine is a menacing superstar on the global illicit-drug stage. Annual South American cocaine production is estimated to exceed 1 million pounds, much of which goes right up the noses, or into the lungs, of U.S. citizens—and has taken the lives of thousands. In other words, coca tea is good for you, but cocaine can kill you. This gives testimony to the fact that tinkering with nature beyond a certain point can prove disastrous.

HEAD-SPLITTING HEIGHTS

Higher up in the mountains, snow began to fall heavy and wet, slowing our progress. The windshield fogged inside, and slushy buildup on the outside taxed the wipers. When we stopped at a small town for a lunch of rellenos with rice and salsa, the air outside the car had a cold bite to it, which conspired with wind and humidity to make a chilling environment. After 9 long, slow hours of driving through altitudes that topped off at more than 16,000 feet at the highest point, we pulled into Cerro de Pasco.

Cerro de Pasco greeted us like an emphysema victim. A grimy mining town with one of the largest open pit mines in the world, Cerro de Pasco boasts the largest population living at the highest altitude anywhere in the world. At almost 15,000 feet, Cerro de Pasco offers bleak terrain, a high incidence of respiratory disorders, and altitude sickness for those who venture up from lower elevations. The town is built around scarified earth, and the people who live there are very poor. Humble mud dwellings and wretched tin shanties line rutted, muddy streets, a scene completed by narrow alleys and mangy dogs. Still, the campesinos were quick with a smile and a wave.

We arrived at a cavernous and cold hotel called the Villa Minera, which advertised both plumbing and electricity. "This is the best place in Cerro de Pasco," Sergio informed us as he rubbed his aching kidneys. The short walk from the Toyota to the front desk made me woozy. But on the way inside I noticed a poster announcing that in just a couple of days, Cerro de Pasco would host the Third Annual National Maca Festival. In fact, the event would take place right across the street from our hotel. Fortune may favor the prepared, but in our case, the coincidental timing of our visit to Cerro and the festival was pure serendipity.

After Shahannah and I checked into our room, I discovered that the toilet didn't flush and that the hot water spigots were purely ornamental. I inquired about the situation with the toilets at the front desk downstairs, and the woman behind the counter told me, "We will turn on the flush water in the morning." Oh. Of course. Our whole crew assembled at a small restaurant nearby for a dinner of chaufa—chicken with rice and a few vegetables. When dinner was over, we returned to the Villa Minera and settled in for a night of hell.

On a hard pallet bed, Shahannah and I found ourselves quickly in the throes of acute altitude sickness. We were short of breath, our hearts were beating rapidly, and both of us succumbed to blinding headaches. We were fatigued, but we couldn't sleep. Shahannah vomited late in the night, and when I wished her happy birthday at 1:00 in the morning, it was nothing but a wan sentiment in a rapidly declining condition.

Also known as mountain sickness, altitude sickness is caused by a lack of oxygen. As altitude increases, atmospheric pressure decreases and fewer oxygen molecules are present in the thin air. To compensate for the atmospheric change, breathing becomes faster and deeper, disrupting the natural balance of gases in the lungs and the blood and altering the balance of potassium and sodium in cells. The lips, nails, and skin take on a slightly bluish tinge known as cyanosis. Most people notice few or none of these changes until they reach between 7,000 and 9,000 feet. How quickly or severely the changes occur depends on how quickly you ascend to a higher altitude. If you don't take time to get acclimated, you can get increasingly sicker as you go to increasingly higher altitudes.

Altitude sickness was a new experience for Shahannah and me. I've climbed more than 16,000 feet in the Sierra Nevada mountain range, but I had never made the mistake of going from sea level to 15,000 feet in one day and then staying overnight. What we should have done was spend a night at 9,000 feet, and then take an additional day for each remaining 2,000 feet, thus allowing our bodies time to become acclimated. In other words, we should have taken 4 days to reach Cerro de Pasco, not 9 hours.

By morning we were both wrung out. I knew we needed to get out of town or risk passing into the more serious phases of altitude sickness, which include pulmonary and cerebral edema. In the former condition, the lungs fill with fluid. In the latter, the brain swells with fluid, leading to a splitting headache, hallucinations, and, possibly, death. Shahannah couldn't walk without assistance, her lips had a bluish tinge, and she was so mentally confused that I figured she was bordering on the real bad stuff. I knocked on Sergio's door around 5:30 A.M. and explained the situation. He, too, had had a bad night, but not as bad as ours. "Yeah, man," he agreed. "We got to go to a lower place. We'll get the truck ready and get out of here."

Outside the hotel, Sergio introduced me to Raúl, who lives in Cerro de Pasco and knows the Central Highlands well. Raúl assists Sergio in the maca trade in the highlands and knows all the growers. Cheerful, strong, and friendly, Raúl would turn out to be a welcome addition to our ever-mutating group. Raúl, Sergio, Shahannah, and I drank some coca tea at the hotel. It warmed us up, but we weren't revived in the least. We packed into the Toyota and drove into town to deposit Rubén at the bus station, so he could head back to Lima. I imagined it would be a pretty rough ride for him, bouncing and charging down mountainsides in one of the scary ghost buses from the 1940s.

In the center of town by the Mercado Municipal, crowds of people milled around shops and stalls. Fruit and vegetable vendors sold colorful papayas, bananas, oranges, onions, herbs, apples, and greens. Boys did brisk business buffing the leather shoes of men and women. It was a vibrant morning scene.

One cart in particular caught my eye. It was run by a woman who was making drinks by mixing herbal extracts from different bottles with liquor-pouring tops, and then adding boiling water from a large, steaming teapot. Shahannah was too sick to get out of the truck, but I went over to the cart and had a drink of alfalfa, coca, boldo (an invigorating South American plant), uña de gato, and boiled water. The drink was hot and tasted pleasant, and I felt a bit picked up after drinking it. I brought a glass back to the truck for Shahannah and plied her with the hot elixir. She lay on her side with the glass to her cyanic lips and slurped. "What is this stuff?" she asked. I explained that it was an herbal drink that might help her to feel a little less woozy.

In fact, the brew served by the woman contained one of the most used plants in the Amazon. Among the many Amazonian botanicals that have come to light in recent years, uña de gato (*Uncaria tomentosa*), which means "cat's claw" in Spanish, is one of the most promising. A woody vine, it earned its name from its sharp, clawlike thorns. Dispersed throughout Central and South America, uña de gato has been used for centuries by numerous native tribes.

Dr. James Duke describes uña de gato in his *Amazonian Ethnobotanical Dictionary* as widely used in Peru for anti-inflammatory, contraceptive, and cytostatic (tumor-cell retarding) purposes. In popular literature, uña de gato is touted as

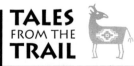

The Cat's Claw

Unlike in Peru, uña de gato remains a minor herb amidst the plethora of supplements on the U.S. market. Nevertheless, you can find and use this amazing Amazon plant as a loose herb and in tablets, capsules, and liquid extracts.

At this point there's no solid science on what a proper dosage might be. Herbalists claim, however, that dosages of up to 7,500 milligrams daily are safe. Common sense should always be your guide, and pregnant or lactating women as well as children under 12 years of age should consult a physician.

If you make a tea of uña de gato, steep 1 tablespoon or so in a quart of boiling water for 5 minutes. Strain, and drink throughout the day as needed.

an immune stimulant. Marketing hype has exaggerated the benefits of this plant, but a number of studies do in fact suggest that uña de gato may be beneficial for anti-inflammatory and immune-enhancing purposes, and that constituents in the vine may help to inhibit tumor cell formation.

Uña de gato first came to the attention of the European scientific community in the early 1970s when Austrian Klaus Keplinger heard of a remarkable cancer cure attributed to the use of the plant. Since that time, researchers have plumbed uña de gato's chemical secrets in search of what might account for its purported healing benefits. Analysis shows that *Uncaria tomentosa* contains at least five alkaloids and two other important groups of compounds—quinovic acid glycosides and triterpenoid saponins. In addition, the plant contains antioxidant polyphenols.

In vitro studies with uña de gato show that certain constituents in the plant possess anti-inflammatory, antimutagenic, antiviral, and immune-stimulating properties. The alkaloids in uña de gato demonstrate immune-enhancing activity by producing an increase in phagocytosis, a process by which potentially harmful materials are "eaten" by protective cells. In studies of the plant's quinovic acid glycosides, researchers observed significant anti-inflammatory activity. These same compounds were shown to inhibit several types of common viruses. And in studying triterpenoid saponins, scientists observed that these chemical agents inhibited the growth of some tumor cells.

While the effective use of beneficial plants existed long before the invention of scientific methods, good scientific studies—such as those that appear to validate several of the traditional uses of uña de gato—provide assurance of herbal efficacy to today's modern, medically oriented market. The plant appears to be safe, nontoxic, and useful in cases of inflammation, compromised immunity, and viral infection. With further research, it may eventually play a role in a complementary approach to the prevention and treatment of certain types of cancer. Meanwhile, tribal people in the Amazon would no doubt be amused by scientific inquiries into uña de gato. They've known for centuries that this plant is a healer.

On the way out of town, we circumnavigated the county-size crater of the Cerro mine. So immense is the crater that the huge mineral trucks that haul from the mine appeared as tiny specks when viewed from the other side. We passed reeking pools of stagnant water as well as several odd monuments to mining. The largest was a pair of hands thrust up from the ground and holding a miner's lantern, as if the rest of the man were buried alive. Another was a faceless, helmeted miner drilling on a piece of stone that so closely resembled a likeness of the Virgin Mary that the effect was one of boring a hole through her forehead. Truly strange.

We dropped onto the expansive Junin Plateau, where lamb and sheep grazed, and where the view stretched for 50 miles. The broad plateau was mostly grassland, with hills and long, inspiring vistas of the great Andes. In sharp contrast to Cerro, the Junin Plateau was splendid to behold and reminded me of parts of Colorado or the great Chama Valley of northern New Mexico. Roaming the valley were llamas and shaggy alpaca. Already I was feeling a bit better, but Shahannah remained in a lethargic, confused state.

In the small highland town of Carhuamayo 45 minutes away, we picked up Enrique, who had come in early on an overnight bus from Lima. He appeared cold and uncomfortable, and seemed happy to climb into the warm truck with its heater on high. Carhuamayo is small, mostly brown in all directions, and filled with low buildings of adobe. We drove down a packed, rutted, very bouncy dirt road and stopped in front of two wooden doors on a faded yellow building. Here we would find a man named César, whom Sergio described as one of the great maca experts in the highlands. "This guy knows everything about maca," he said. "He helps many, many people to grow maca and to be sure that they get a good crop. He is one of the best people involved in the maca scene up here." César greeted us at the door and welcomed us with a firm handshake.

Inside, storage bags of dried maca filled a large front room with a concrete floor. Some of the maca roots were large, some small. I was surprised that some were yellow and others purple, and said so. "Oh, yes," César responded. "Maca grows in several colors. People in the highlands prefer the cream-colored roots, although the Germans want black roots. As far as we know, there is no significant difference between colors of roots and health benefits. But that is probably something to look into."

César described the importance of drying maca. "If you are going to preserve maca, you must dry it correctly," he said. "It takes up to 1 year to fully dry the roots." He picked up two maca roots, one noticeably more shriveled and compact than the other. He handed the shriveled one to me and said, "Press your thumbnail into this one." I tried, but the root was like a small rock, hard and unyielding. "That root is fully dry." César smiled and handed me the other. "But try this one." I pushed my thumbnail into the less shriveled root, and it made a noticeable indentation. "This root has been drying for several months," César said. "But it will have to dry for several more. The roots require cool and dry conditions. If they get wet, they will spoil. Most people who grow maca will dry the roots in the sun for a few weeks, and after that the roots are stored inside in a protected place with enough air to circulate and keep them drying."

César, we were informed, would join us later in Cerro de Pasco at the maca festival. The rest of us headed for the town of Yanahuanca, 2 hours away and, at 6,000 feet, safely out of the altitude-sickness zone. The road to Yanahuanca took us from the thin air of the Junín Plateau steadily down long, winding roads to a warmer and much more scenic Peru. Sergio rubbed his aching kidneys. "You know, I'm glad we're coming down here," he confessed.

Shiny blue eucalyptus trees stood together in dense stands alongside the roads and covered much of the hills. Their fragrant terpene aroma brightened my senses and opened my lungs. It felt good to breathe deeply, taking in a richer mix of oxygen. Huge agave with thick, spearlike leaves grew profusely, standing proudly from even the steepest slopes. Around one curve, we spotted a bald eagle. The majestic raptor flew low and close, then tipped a wing and was quickly carried up and away by invisible currents. Soon after, we saw another, then one more.

Finally, we spied in the distance a town nestled deep in the bottom of a valley, surrounded on all sides by steep, terraced peaks. "That's Yanahuanca," Sergio said, pointing. "That's where we're going to stay tonight." Before too long, we pulled into the central plaza of quaint Yanahuanca, with its slow pace, friendly atmosphere, and pretty scenery. Our first order of business was lunch, which we found at Restaurant Pamela, a small, crowded eatery on the plaza. We drank coca tea, ate chaufa, and relaxed in an atmosphere in which we could breathe comfortably and get around without feeling dizzy.

That afternoon we visited a hot spring, where we could bathe and recuperate. Outside the small bath house, women sold soap, crackers, and candy. Children played in a pool fed by the hot springs, laughing and screaming as they jumped into the slightly yellow, sulfuric water, deriving endless pleasure from splashing each other. When it was our turn to bathe, a man in rubber boots led us into a small tiled room and showed us how to control the scalding hot and frigid waters that ran into the tub area. Both flowed at fire-hose force from holes in the wall unless they were stopped up, which was accomplished by inserting fat wooden plugs. The bath was fantastic, and we cooked ourselves in the aromatic, mineralized waters until we were squeaky clean and flushed red.

Outside, the rubber-booted attendant asked if we wanted to see where the springs came from the ground. We followed him behind the bath house to a natural pool that bubbled and steamed and smelled of minerals. I dipped a fingertip into the water and discovered that at its source it was nearly boiling. A few yards away, a cold stream flowed. Manmade troughs diverted the hot and cold waters into the baths, and it was all very simple. I gave the man two *nuevos soles*, and he was appreciative.

By the end of the afternoon, I felt back to normal, and Shahannah was getting there. That night we slept in a cramped room whose shower stall had a floor covered with viscous goo, and whose bathroom sink drained directly onto the floor. The whole place smelled of urine, but we passed into deep sleep, barely noticing the atrocious condition of our lodging.

The next day, we took our time with breakfast at Restaurant Pamela, as if to delay the unwelcome drive back to evil Cerro de Pasco. Sergio was confident that after our stay in Yanahuanca, we'd be all right staying at the Villa Minera that night. I wasn't so sure.

After arriving in Cerro, we picked up Techi, Masha, and Amy, who had come in on the overnight bus from Lima. Following a roiling hailstorm, we sat in the sun in front of Villa Minera with a plant geneticist named Dante, who has devoted the last several years of his career to the study of maca. Although we talked about little that was extraordinary, the circumstance of the conversation was remarkable—and hard to explain. Dante spoke only in Spanish, a language with which I am minimally familiar and have never studied. I can ask for beer and bathrooms, know the names of a few foods, and can say *adiós*. Yet, though Dante was describing in very scientific and technical Spanish some of the finer points of his genetic research into maca, I somehow was able to follow almost every word. Even stranger, I was able, in that conversation alone, to ask technical questions in passable Spanish. Sergio and César noticed this, and they looked at me with heads cocked, wondering what the heck was going on.

Dante spoke about what César had touched on back in Carhuamayo—that maca grows in several colors. Dante believes that each color is a "pure genetic strain." Exactly how this color differentiation came about is not certain. Nor can maca growers yet purchase batches of seeds that produce roots of specific colors. "When growers acquire seeds, they are all mixed," he explained. "Thus a maca plot will yield roots of several colors—red, green, black, purple, cream. Geneticists are working to collect and separate seeds from specific colored roots. Once they have enough of each one, cultivation of specific colored roots can be more easily accomplished." Such color-specific cultivation, Dante went on, will enable researchers to more carefully study whether or not there are any significant chemical differences between pure-colored strains. If, for example, black (*negro*) maca is higher in isothiocyanates than other colors, then that color maca might be grown in greater quantity than other colors.

After a couple of hours in the warm sun, we broke for lunch and coca tea. I was wondering about the linguistic mind-meld we'd just had, and so was Sergio. "Hey, what happened out there with you and Dante?" he asked. "That was pretty cool, man." We shook hands and laughed. These kinds of things can and do happen on the road, providing a certain element of curiosity and a mystical tinge to whatever experience is occurring. After that conversation, I went from my temporary fluency to being a non–Spanish-speaking person once again.

SPIRITS, THUNDER, AND LIGHTNING

Late that afternoon, Sergio, Dante, César, Enrique, Shahannah, Raúl, and I piled into the Toyota and another pickup truck and hurried out of Cerro De Pasco to Ninagaga, a small highland town where Sergio had purchased land to build a maca center. We were headed there so Enrique could perform a shamanic purification ritual to bless the land and propitiate the spirits. When we got to the town, a sign on the road said Ninacaca, not Ninagaga. I pointed this out, and Sergio laughed, "Oh yeah, they put up that sign that says *caca*, because, you know, they think this town is crap. But the name really is Ninagaga." Shahannah and I cracked up.

By the time we all arrived at Sergio's land in Ninagaga, the sun was setting and a cold wind was coming up. Once we were out of our trucks and into the center of Sergio's field, Enrique piled together twigs and boards for a fire, which we got going with the help of a liberal dosing of gasoline. The fire lit, Enrique set up an altar on the ground, replete with artifacts of various kinds, including a small wooden sword, some polished sticks, crystals, a ceramic pyramid, a woven medicine bag, a small satchel of coca leaves, and figurines of deities from the Christian, Hindu, Buddhist, and Egyptian traditions. Enrique opened a bottle of high-octane *pisco* and poured a small amount in a cup. He drank some and threw some at the fire as he chanted softly to himself. Enrique removed his jacket and rolled up his shirt sleeves. The rest of us were cold against a bitter wind, and we huddled as close to the fire as possible.

While Enrique was preparing for the ceremony, two men came across the field toward us. One had a raw, elemental look and feel about him, as though he had just walked in from some other wild dimension. He moved a bit like a coyote. Something about him made the hair on the back of my neck prickle. Even though the sky was heavy with ponderous charcoal clouds and the last light of day was fast slipping into black, the man wore dark sunglasses. The two men looked briefly at our pitifully small fire and slipped away after a few muttered words. A few moments later they returned with huge armloads of freshly cut straw, a great pile of which they added to the fire. The fire crackled and sprang high with leaping flames, moving us back from its edge. The two men drifted off without saying a word, and we never saw them again.

Enrique began to chant, calling out to the gods and spirits. He chewed a large quid of coca leaf and splashed *pisco* around. Then he produced a well-tied package about the size of a loaf of bread and placed it in the fire. He poured more *pisco*, drank some, sprinkled some on the fire, and splashed some more around. The package burned slowly, and Enrique waved his arms about and called to the spirits. Thunder boomed and lightning flashed in sky-splitting streaks. The neatly tied package was consumed in flames.

Then Enrique poured some amber crystals onto the fire. The crystals sparked and the aroma rose like pungent church incense. As all seven of us stood around the fire, Enrique began to offer psychic information to each of us, beginning with Shahannah. He told her that she had an excellent perception of the spirits, and the soul of a warrior. He said that she carried with her the power of her Cherokee heritage. She would find a surprise when she got home, and she would be especially pleased in her family life and her work. Shahannah gave Enrique a piece of meteoric glass, and as the wind blew freezing and the night sky roiled with thunder and flashed with lightning, Enrique returned the offering with a polished hardwood sword, which he presented with a courteous bow.

When Enrique got to me he said that I was very good at ideas and healthy living, and that things would go extremely well for me in my pursuit to popularize natural medicines. I offered Enrique a jaguar's tooth I'd been wearing on a cord around my neck, and he gave me in return a peculiar white porcelain pyramid with Isis on one side.

Enrique gave specific insights to each person in the group, extending wishes for blessings from the spirits. Then he put some more straw on the fire, splashed some more *pisco* around, drank some more of it, and declared the purification ritual for the Ninagaga maca center complete. Barely had that declaration been uttered when the sky boomed with bomblike thunder, the wind rose to a howling intensity, and a driving rain blew down upon us with such sudden force that we were sent scrambling in the dark back to our trucks.

Enrique's shamanic ceremony at Ninagaga was intended to imbue Sergio's maca center with sacred energy. The appearance of the two strange men, and the impeccable timing of the weather, gave a primal, otherworldly potency to the event. It was as if the spirits, in cooperation with Enrique, were moving things along in a wild and magical way.

A FEAST OF MACA

Back at the Villa Minera, we had another horrible night, though not as bad as the first. "I will never sleep in this town again," Shahannah declared the next morning. "I don't care what we have to do, but I will never spend another night here in my life." I couldn't really argue with her. After coca tea we went to a clinic for oxygen along with Sergio, Techi, Masha, and Amy, all of whom had also suffered through a wretched night. Both Shahannah and I wished we had known previously that oxygen was available in Cerro de Pasco. At the clinic, while locals were being examined for cuts, sprains, and other health conditions, we lay on beds with tubes up our noses, taking in the cool, gaseous stream, which helped to revive us and back us away from the edge of more serious complications. The infusion of oxygen helped to get our brains functioning for the Third Annual National Maca Festival.

By midmorning, the grassy fairgrounds in Cerro were a bustling enclave of tents, tarps, and tabletops, with displays of every conceivable aspect of maca cultivation and processing. Plastic banners and flags proclaimed "Maca!" Shahannah and I were pretty much inured to being stared at in the Central Highlands. But as the only two gringos at the maca festival, we drew from the very start a curious retinue of young boys, teenage girls, and assorted adults trailing behind us wherever we went, wanting to see what we were looking at, eager to observe our reactions to what we tried, and either dashing away from our cameras or jockeying for advantage in front of them. "You're going to be an attraction all to yourselves," Sergio told us.

One side of the fair was oriented mostly toward maca agriculture. Several booths displayed the many colors of maca roots, some with signs labeling their colors. A few exhibited broad, seed-bearing maca flowers, and some maca growers demonstrated how the seeds are shaken out of their pods, then screened and cleaned, yielding ready-to-plant maca seed for the next year's planting. A few maca growers displayed healthy maca plants in small ceramic pots. If we wanted to, we could have purchased a few pounds of maca seed right then and there to start our own highland plots.

The growers were surprised to see us and asked why we were there. When we explained that maca was a plant likely to become popular in the United States, they were obviously proud, and they took our interest as a positive sign. "It is the very best plant in the world," one grower stated flatly.

More tempting to Shahannah and me were the booths and tables displaying maca food products. Several exhibitors offered bags of maca flour ready for use in baking. One man stood beside a large display of nicely packaged maca cookies. "Are they any good?" I inquired. He offered me a cookie, and to my pleasant surprise it tasted pretty much like a well-made graham cracker, but denser and crunchier. The man smiled and told us that he practiced yoga regularly, and that maca was an impor-

Making maca blender drinks at a maca festival

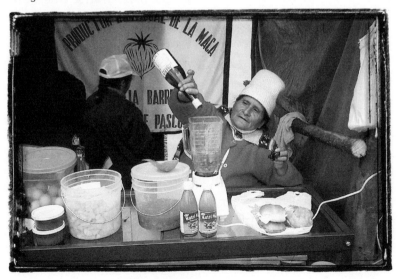

tant part of his vitality program. I bought 10 bags of cookies, giving some to Sergio, and we moved along on a slow sampling journey that would leave us stuffed by late afternoon.

At several booths, maca roots were soaking in jars of water, and the tables were laden with ingredients for maca blender drinks. The typical shake included a couple of soaked maca roots and a little bit of the soak water, a handful of fresh papaya trucked up from the warm lowlands, some condensed milk, an egg, honey, and vanilla—all put together with vigor and smiles from the women who made them. Tasting one blender drink meant being obliged to taste them all. Every woman making blender drinks assured us that while the other women at the fair made good drinks, hers was surely the best. "You will see for yourself," one woman confided. "The other drinks are okay, but when you taste mine, then you will understand the real maca drink." We stopped at six or seven booths, sampling the blender drinks made at each one. They were all good.

Along the way, I shot stills and Shahannah shot video. Our photographic efforts were such a disrupting fascination to the Peruvians that it was hard to navigate through the throng of interested onlookers crowded around us. As we pointed our cameras in various directions, young boys jostled and elbowed each other as they crowded into a shot, while teenage girls giggled, put their hands to their faces, and fled. Most of the women making the blender drinks expected us to photograph them, and they posed proudly with their ingredients and appliances.

At one booth I encountered a big, bubbling pot of mazzamora, a popular highland porridge made of maca, the Andean grains quinoa and kiwicha, eggs, milk, honey, and vanilla. A stocky woman ladled up a big bowl for me. I can power my way through a lot of food, but I was beginning to wonder how I would make it through the whole fair. To my delight, the porridge was really good stuff, something I could eat every morning.

On the somewhat more unusual side, we encountered maca Jell-O and maca flan. Both, as it turned out, were surprisingly

Maca Shakes

I am a maca user, not just an observer or commentator. Here are two of my favorite maca blender drink recipes. After drinking either one, I can breeze through hours of intense work without flagging or losing concentration.

The Junin Shake

Something between a shake and a meal, the Junin Shake is the way maca blender drinks are made in the Peru's Junin Plateau, where maca grows. The papaya, of course, comes from down in the lowlands. Simply blend the following until smooth.

1 handful of fresh papaya

4 ounces of water

1 tablespoon of powdered maca

About 3 ounces of condensed milk (you can use whole milk)

1 raw egg (organic, of course)

Honey, to taste

Vanilla extract, to taste

Medicine Hunter Maca Drink

This is my own recipe, and it works great. Again, blend the following until smooth.

8 ounces of papaya, pear, or apple juice (organic is always best)

2 tablespoons of vanilla yogurt

1 ripe banana

1 tablespoon of powdered maca

Vanilla extract, to taste

good. Several women made maca marmalade, which they sold in small plastic deli tubs, just the way you get slaw and potato salad at a store. At one booth, a man and woman were producing maca chips in a little fryolator as fast as they could—and people were scarfing them up even faster. The chips were light and porous, like the rice chips served in some Chinese restaurants.

We discovered several kinds of bottled maca products, including sweet maca syrup, juices with maca, and maca liquor. Shahannah and I agreed to be careful with the liquor, especially at the high altitude. But our mutual warnings and best intentions were useless. In no time at all, we were sucked into a vortex of maca liquor samples that were coming at us fast and furious from all directions. Every maker of maca liquor assured us that theirs was the very best—and plied us with delicious drinks to prove it. We both got a little plotzed. At one point, a man walked up to me with a twisted grin, thrust a bottle at me, and encouraged me to drink. I took a sip of what can only be described as maca-flavored firewater. The man gave me a crooked, toothless smile, nodded his head up and down as though we'd just shared a special secret, and melted back into the crowd. Ah, the hazards of rigorous field research.

Just about when I figured we'd had all we could take of maca products, the judging began for the maca baking competition. We weren't judges, but we were herded over to a long expanse of baker's tables and given multiple pieces of cake. Even though our opinions made no difference in the outcome of the competition, all eyes turned to us as we sampled one cake after another. Even as we were tasting one piece of cake, the bakers, all women, would thrust others at us, making comments like, "Mine is better, you will see." Shahannah got off easy with

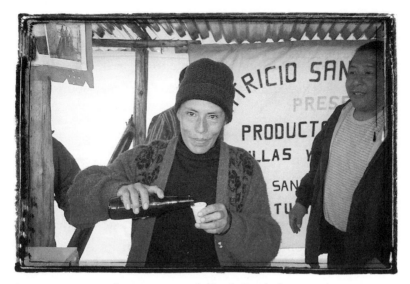

A woman pours maca liquor as maca trader Sergio Cam looks on

smaller pieces, but I was given great fat wedges of every cake, all good. I mmmed and ahhhed and smacked my lips through each piece, silently praying that there wasn't a maca pie contest to follow. As we walked away from the cake tables, Shahannah leaned up against me. "I don't think I can eat much more maca today," she confided.

We spent the entire afternoon at the Third Annual National Maca Festival, passed the night at the comfortable Huanuco Hotel at a lower altitude, and returned to Cerro for another day at the festival. We talked with vendors, sampled all the maca products yet again, took photographs, and shot video. I asked one couple who had just purchased maca blender drinks why they used maca. "Well, for energy, of course," the woman answered, "but it's very good for sex." She smiled, blushing, and rubbed her shoulder against her partner.

The maca festival drew to a close. Stuffed beyond capacity

from sampling, all of us were glad to get out of Cerro de Pasco. It may be the center of maca trade in the Central Highlands, but the place was just too uncomfortable to linger in. We squeezed like anchovies into the Toyota and made the long, laborious trip back to Lima.

Maca is being studied by eminent scientists worldwide. As it has become increasingly well-known, its use has spread to medical practices. The November, 1998 issue of the *Townsend Letter for Doctors* quoted several physicians regarding the therapeutic and salutary uses of maca. Hugo Malaspina, M.D., a cardiologist practicing complementary medicine in Lima, has been using maca in his practice for 10 years. He commonly recommends maca to women experiencing premenstrual discomfort or menopausal symptoms, because of its regulating effects on the ovaries and other internal organs. "I have had perhaps 200 female patients whose perimenopausal and menopausal symptoms were alleviated by taking maca," Dr. Malaspina said.

Aguila Calderon, M.D., the former dean of the faculty of human medicine at the National University of Federico Villarreal in Lima, commented on the relationship between maca's uses and its mineral value. "Maca has a lot of easily absorbable calcium in it, plus magnesium, and a fair amount of silica, which we are finding very useful in treating the decalcification of bones in children and adults," he said. In his practice, Dr. Calderon uses maca for erectile dysfunction, menopausal symptoms, and general fatigue.

Will maca become a popular, widely consumed herb in the United States? I think it has a good shot at that status. After all, it safely and effectively enhances both energy and sex, and almost everybody wants to enhance one or the other or both. A good indication of the future is the way a January, 1999 article in the *Miami Herald* described maca as "Peru's natural Viagra." Once a reporter from the *Wall Street Journal* asked me what it takes for an herb to become popular. My answer was, "You." In a media-driven culture, it takes the enthusiasm and support of the media to bring herbs to the attention of the mainstream public.

I believe such enthusiastic media attention will turn increasingly to maca for all the right reasons. As more people turn to natural products for safer alternatives to potentially dangerous drugs, and as more people realize that nature does indeed provide vitality-enhancing superfoods, maca may just be a future herbal superstar waiting for its time in the spotlight.

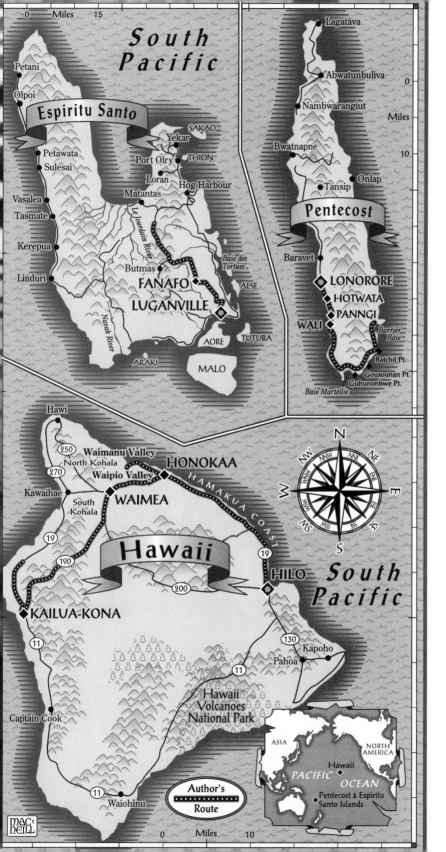

South Pacific

Espiritu Santo

Petani
Olpoi
Petawata
Sulesai
Vasalea
Tasmate
Kerepua
Linduri
Yekar
SAKAO
Port Olry
THION
Loran
Matantas
Hog Harbour
Le Jourdain River
Baie des Tortues
Butmas
FANAFO
AESE
LUGANVILLE
Navak River
AORE
ARAKI
TUTUBA
MALO

Lagatava
Abwatunbuliva
Nambwarangiut
Bwatnapne
Onlap
Tansip
Pentecost
Baravet
LONORORE
HOTWATA
PANNGI
WALI
Barrier Baie
Batchil Pt.
Gousounan Pt.
Guhunonbwe Pt.
Baie Martellie

Hawi
250
Waimanu Valley
North Kohala
270
Waipio Valley
HONOKAA
HAMAKUA COAST
Kawaihae
WAIMEA
South Kohala
19
Hawaii
19
190
HILO
South Pacific
200
KAILUA-KONA
11
11
Hawaii Volcanoes National Park
130
Kapoho
Pahoa
Captain Cook
11
Waiohinu

Author's Route

Miles 0 — 10

ASIA
NORTH AMERICA
Hawaii
PACIFIC OCEAN
Pentecost & Espiritu Santo Islands

MACt NEILL

Nights of Kava

FRAGRANT HILL

As we rolled past the forests of the Hamakua coast of the Big Island of Hawaii, Zachary Gibson hugged his large Polynesian body close to the steering wheel of his supercharged Dodge Ram pickup and shared random thoughts with me on water safety for the short boat ride we were about to take. "I don't really worry too much about what to do out on the water. I mean, I basically know how to handle most situations out there," he said. "Let's say for example that the boat flips over in the waves. Then what you do is leave all the gear and swim to shore. Now if you get caught in a bad situation like that out by the cliffs, then sure, you probably wouldn't make it. So, well, you just try not to wind up in that situation."

As Zachary delivered this less than reassuring monologue, his wife Hanna and her niece Margaret shared space in the bed of the truck with a large cooler, gear bags, tents, food, and all the gear we needed to camp out for a few days. Behind the truck, an inflated, hard-rubber Zodiac—the kind of hardy watercraft favored by ocean researchers and environmental action groups for navigating bumpy seas—bounced along on its trailer.

Zack slowly crept the truck down a steep paved road etched into the side of the verdant Waipio Valley, one of several huge valleys in the northernmost Kohala district of Hawaii. Nestled like glistening emeralds in the Kohala Forest Reserve, and carved back into the crenelated volcanic Kohala Mountains, the Waipio Valley and the nearby Waimanu Valley boast some of the most spectacular scenery in Hawaii—and a rich diversity of exciting plant life.

A former San Francisco chef turned certified organic kava farmer, Zachary is a true Hawaiian cowboy, shooting wild pigs from on top of a horse, fishing the rivers and ocean, hiking the forests and valleys, and bodysurfing. "I'm totally insane in the waves," he confessed. Over the past several years, he had been exploring the Waipio and Waimanu Valleys for old kava plants, an herb well-known for its ability to quell anxiety. Two years earlier, Zachary and some other friends and I had hiked deep into the Waipio Valley, with its dozens of waterfalls twisting down the sides of steep cliffs several hundred feet high. There we edged along narrow trails of loose volcanic scree high up on the hillsides to reach a planting of giant kava the size of trees, more than 20 feet high with limbs thick enough to hang from.

But this time we'd be going up the even more remote Waimanu Valley, accessible only by a day-long hike or, in our case, by boat. We planned to launch from the river mouth of the Waipio, go out past the waves, head north along the coast, and beach the boat at the mouth of the Waimanu, where we would set up camp. The next day, Zack and I would hike deep into the valley in search of kava plants.

This trip to Hawaii was an important one for my ongoing research into kava, from its role in Pacific island cultures to its commerce in the United States and throughout the world. Hawaii itself is at something of a kava crossroads. While its current participation in the burgeoning kava trade is modest, a number of growers in the Hawaiian Islands are taking steps to become big suppliers. I was there to meet them, learn about their plans, and examine their cultivation efforts firsthand. The information would get me up-to-date on this aspect of the kava trade, and help me in my capacity as advisor to companies involved with or interested in kava. And for a historical perspective, I wanted to get into at least one more of the sacred valleys on the Big Island to see for myself some old strands of kava left over from traditional native planters from another era.

KAVA, THE PEACE ELIXIR

The kava plant is an esteemed mind- and mood-altering agent that occupies a central place in culture and custom throughout Oceania, the large geographic area in the South Pacific ranging from Hawaii and the Marianas Islands along the Tropic of Cancer down to New Zealand below the Tropic of Capricorn. Oceania includes three distinct cultural regions—Polynesia, Melanesia, and Micronesia—and offers some of the most exotic island life on Earth. The swaying palm trees, volcanic landscapes, glistening sandy beaches, vast coral reefs, and indigenous native cultures of Oceania represent a notion of paradise widely held among peoples of other parts of the world.

Kava refers both to the plant *Piper methysticum* and to a pungent beverage prepared from its roots. A robust and attractive perennial shrub with smooth, heart-shaped green leaves, kava is a member of the *Piperaceae*, or pepper, family. At least 2,000 species have been widely distributed since antiquity throughout Africa, India, Southeast Asia, and Indonesia. A small number of *Piper* species are used as spices and medicines, including *Piper nigrum*, from whose red berries both black and white peppercorns are prepared, and *Piper betle*, whose nut contains a stimulant known as arecoline. The nut is chewed with lime throughout much of Southeast Asia.

Piper methysticum, or cultivated kava, is a descendant of wild kava, *Piper wichmannii*. Botanists assert that at one time all kava was *Piper wichmannii*. But cultivated kava is greatly preferred over wild kava, which is only rarely used as an "extender" when cultivated kava is in short supply. A lush, leafy green plant, kava grows densely and is harvested when it is approximately 6 to 8 feet in height and 5 to 7 years old. At that age, kava roots have typically become a thick, knotted mass and are suitable for the preparation of the kava beverage.

Today numerous varieties of kava are cultivated, distinguished by their physical characteristics and by their effects upon body and mind. The relative proportions and potencies of the active constituents from one variety to another determine the nature and intensity of the psychosomatic effects. Some varieties of kava are considered ideal for drinking. These preferred varieties act very quickly, produce a significant relaxing and tranquilizing effect, and leave no dullness or hangover.

In some island cultures the consumption of kava was largely the privilege of chiefs and men of high rank. Such strict social delineation has diminished over time, but status still plays an important role in kava consumption. Whoever ranks highest at a kava ceremony is served first, and the rest are served in order of their social standing. Ambassadors, dignitaries, and officials from other nations are regularly served kava when they visit or hold important meetings on South Pacific islands. Kava con-

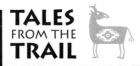
The Kava Effect: Do It Right

Kava is nature's Valium without the side effects. When made into the right extract and consumed in the right amount, kava can relieve stress, quell anxiety, and help even the most fitful sleeper enjoy a night of peaceful rest. Is it any surprise that its popularity in the United States has skyrocketed in recent years?

As a result of the explosion in its popularity, you'll find a plethora of kava products on the market. Unfortunately, many of them are useless. Any product that contains only ground-up kava root—either in tablets or in capsules—is a total waste. You simply cannot eat enough ground-up kava root to get any benefit. Only kava extracts, either in powder or liquid form, will deliver the kava effect you want.

You can indeed find such extracts in tablets and capsules. But don't bother with a kava product unless it explicitly states on the label that it contains at least 70 milligrams of kavalactones per dose. This is the bare minimum effective dose as established in clinical trials.

Better yet are fluid kava extracts. Short of packing off to a Pacific island, they're the closest you're likely to get to the real time-honored kava experience. You'll find lots of them in natural food stores, and I list some of my favorite brands in Resources on page 281. But I also have some recommendations on what to do with the liquid kava extract once you get it home.

First, arrange the company of a friend; kava is a social substance. Take it on an empty stomach. Pour a full teaspoon of liquid kava extract into a cup (a paper cup is better because it's hard to get kava residue off a glass). Add a couple of ounces of water. Slug it down—all of it—immediately. Your tongue will numb for a couple of minutes, and then you'll feel the wave of the kava effect. Wait about 25 minutes before having a second cup.

I think you'll agree with me that kava is a fabulous plant with effects that are as pleasant as they are beneficial.

sumption is integral to life in that region, and it's the first act at important traditional community functions and gatherings.

Though kava's primary use throughout Oceania is as a social, mood-enhancing beverage, the plant is also part of the native pharmacopoeia of the region and is used medicinally for a wide range of conditions. The primary folk medicinal use of kava is for urogenital inflammation and cystitis. But kava is also drunk to relieve headaches, to restore vigor, to promote urination, to soothe an unruly stomach, to relieve whooping cough in children, and to ameliorate symptoms of asthma and tuberculosis. Applied topically, kava is useful for treating fungal infections and for soothing stings and skin inflammations.

Kava is also prized for its ornamental and spiritual worth. It is central to the rituals and various life passages of the people of Oceania. Thus kava plants are exchanged and used at virtually all significant occasions and ceremonies. Kava plants are often cultivated to grow in specific shapes, and kava plants presented as gifts at weddings and other special occasions are typically decorated.

In Hawaii, cultivated kava is called awa, a name that accompanied the plant when it was brought to Hawaii by Polynesians migrating from the Marquesas Islands around 300 A.D. They also brought banana, breadfruit, coconut, sago palm, sugar cane, ginger, yams, turmeric, sweet potato, and taro. In Hawaiian legend, however, the gods Kane and Kanaloa, not Polynesian voyagers, are credited with first planting awa.

Awa was part of traditional Hawaiian life. The drink made from the pounded roots of the awa plant was used in ceremonial rituals and celebrations, and as a social libation. In contrast to the islands of Samoa, Tonga, or Fiji, where awa was drunk primarily by the elite, in Hawaii the beverage was consumed by all, not just the ali'i (chiefs). Traditional preparation of the awa drink was a time-consuming labor assigned to children, whose teeth were strong enough to masticate the fibrous roots of the plant into a paste. This paste was placed in a calabash called a kanoa, water was added and mixed with the masticated root, and the resulting infusion was strained and drunk.

Kava cultivation not only keeps growers and their friends and communities well supplied with kava, but it's part of a lucrative agricultural enterprise ranging over thousands of miles of South Pacific territory. An increasing amount of kava is now grown for American, French, and German botanical extraction companies that have stepped up their production of kava extracts because of the increased interest in kava's beneficial effects. In Hawaii, cultivated kava, or awa, is making a resurgence after being relegated to a cultural relic for decades. In 1893, 17,000 pounds of dried root were exported from Hawaii to Europe and processed into medications for nervous disorders, bladder infections, and menstrual discomfort. Today, Hawaii is starting its awa production and sales all over again.

I was first introduced to kava in 1980 by my herbalist friend Andrew Miller, who always seemed to be carrying around samples of new or little-known botanical products. I grew increasingly fascinated with it over the next few years. In 1995, this interest led me to the islands of Vanuatu, a remote archipelago in the South Pacific believed to be the origin of kava. There I met numerous native kava experts, participated in kava rituals, and became acquainted with the important status that the plant and the beverage made from it occupied in those islands. In the course of my research in Vanuatu, I was made an honorary chief by the people of a small village named Baie Martellie, and eventually I was appointed the consular representative of the Independent Republic of Vanuatu to the United States.

The investigation of medicinal plants can lead to exotic places, talented people, and unusual circumstances. And since plants are central to native cultures, a foray into the world of native plants is a foray into native culture. Many native people maintain that plants are volitional, and they reach out to us. I am inclined to accept this. In the case of kava, the plant definitely seemed to reach out to me, and the result has been a rich journey.

The first time I met Zachary Gibson and his parents Bill and Kahala Ann, we were at a natural products convention in Nashville, Tennessee. Over time we became friends. I respected Zachary's efforts at organic kava farming—a hard trade in the best of circumstances—and admired his exploration of the traditional plantings of the Hawaiians. Half Hawaiian himself, Zachary readily carved out a place in the culture of the Big Island, and he won the respect of other Hawaiians through hard work, successful awa farming, and an expert knowledge of hunting, fishing, boating, riding, and field skills. Zachary was the ideal companion for a hike into the remote reaches of the Waimanu Valley in search of awa.

In 1833, the Waimanu Valley was inhabited by some 2,000 Hawaiians. By 1964, the number had dwindled to 17. Today the Waimanu Valley is an uninhabited forest reserve, with permits issued to a small number of campers. But when the valley was a thriving community, awa was planted abundantly. Zachary had come upon awa while exploring in the Waimanu Valley, but he knew there was more to be seen. "I've been back in there a couple of times," he told me. "But I think that if we go even farther than where I've gone before, we'll find a lot more awa." Zack had spent a few weeks preparing for our Waimanu trip. "I reconditioned the boat," he said. "Plus I've hidden a small aluminum boat there, so we'll be able to row up into the valley instead of hiking the whole way."

After loading up the Zodiac down by the river at Waipio, Zack, Hanna, Margaret, and I donned our life jackets and walked the boat to where the mouth of the river met the beach. When Zack determined that the wave sets were small enough to allow passage out to sea, we piled hurriedly into the boat. Zack started the outboard engine with a quick yank of the cord, pulled the throttle wide open, and roared the boat into the waves. Water smashed us in the faces in great sheets. Just outside of a large set of waves, the engine died. "Oh, God, I can't believe this," Zack wailed, arms in the air. Leaping over the cooler to the outboard, he ripped off the top of the motor, frantically searching for the cause of the engine's demise. We had just a couple of minutes before we'd need to abandon the boat and all our goods, and battle back to shore in pounding surf. I smiled. Zack quickly determined that the fuel line had accidentally disconnected. With fuel supply re-established and the engine primed, we roared off into the rollicking swells of the windswept north coast of Hawaii. "Yeah, that was a little close," Zack shouted over the din of the motor. "But not to worry. We're on our way. We're going to have a great time."

Racing the Zodiac like a Greenpeace rescue boat in a high-speed chase, Zack flew across the tops of big swells as we headed north along high, rocky cliffs. Hanna, Margaret, and I gripped the rail ropes tightly as the boat banged and smashed hard on the surface of the water, like a piano skipping across heaved pavement. "Isn't this great?" Zack called out exuberantly, as he launched us off the top of a large swell into the air. We landed with a crash and spun in a trough before another large swell. "Whoa! Yeehah!" Zack kept the throttle of the Zodiac wide open, and we raced and banged toward the Waimanu Valley. After this jolting thrill ride, we glided to shore on waves that deposited us gently on a rocky beach. There we unpacked the boat, selected a campsite, and put up our tents.

The next morning, Zachary set about making coffee in a battered aluminum pot over a campfire. "I know you like coffee, so I got these Folger bags," he said. "I figure if I use the whole box, it might make a strong-enough pot." Minutes later, we drank the imponderable brew and ate a panful of scrambled eggs and half a loaf of toast. After stuffing four peanut butter and jelly sandwiches into our packs, Zack and I readied ourselves for a day of hiking deep into the forest. Hanna and Margaret had other plans. They intended to take a short, relaxing walk to a large waterfall to swim and sun themselves. "We're going to take it easy while you guys kill yourselves," Hanna joked.

The first order of business was to wade into high, thick grass near the Waimanu River, where Zachary had stashed the aluminum boat he named the Sovereign Queen. "I figure since I'm Hawaiian and I'm totally respectful of the environment, it's okay to keep the boat here," he said. We struggled to get the craft out of its hiding spot, righted it, and set it into the water. "This will save us a lot of hiking time," Zachary explained. "We'll take this as far as we can up the river, and then when the water gets too shallow, we'll tie up and head farther in from there. We'll be able to go a much longer distance this way."

We put into the river with its gentle current and undisturbed surface. Paddling easily, we rounded a long, sweeping curve of high grass and steadily moved up-water toward the back of the expansive valley. To the north, waterfalls twisted down long rocky cliffs and dove into dense foliage. Ahead in the distance, one of the scarred Kohala mountains rose up from a valley floor of brilliant green, and thrust the sharp ridge of its slate-colored peak into a ponderous, misty cloud.

We paddled for three-quarters of an hour, and when the water became shallow, we tied the Sovereign Queen to a tree at the river's edge, grabbed our packs, and set off into dense woods. Right away we came upon a group of ohia'a'ai (*Syzygium malaccense*) trees, also known as mountain apple, hanging heavy with ripe fruit. Throwing down our packs, we pulled the branches low and picked as much as we thought we could eat for the next couple of days. The succulent fruit tasted sweet and juicy, and I ate at least a dozen before packing twice as many more.

Resuming our hike, we passed numerous tall ironwood (*Casuarina equisetifolia*), or toa, with their slender, pine needle–like branchlets. Kiawe (*Prosopis pallida*), with their bright yellow blossoms and sharp thorns, caught our shirts and pants and made razor-fine cuts on our legs. Purple morning glory (*Ipomoea indica*) crept up bushes and radiated color in the glistening sun. Bright orange montbretia (*Crocosmia pottsii*) flowers sat atop tall stalks. Liana of frizzy, white-petaled passion fruit (*Passiflora edulis*) strung themselves like Christmas ornaments across bushes and shrubs. We waded into several large patches of profusely prickly thimbleberry (*Rubus rosifolius*) to capture their sweet, juicy, raspberry-like fruit. Early on in our search for awa, we were well-fed by fruit, and our legs bore tiny cuts in hundreds of places.

In an area of leafy ferns we came upon numerous awapuhi (*Zingiber zerumbet*). Zachary stopped and squeezed a blossom head, and a flush of slippery juice ran into his hand. "See, this is great traditional shampoo," he commented. Brought to Hawaii by Polynesians, awapuhi concentrates in dry, shady areas. When squeezed, the pinecone-like flowering head of the plant yields a volume of silken liquid that makes an excellent shampoo ingredient. Widely cultivated by traditional Hawaiians, awapuhi now grows profusely in the wild and is the dominant plant in some areas. In traditional medicine, underground stems of the plant were rubbed on the scalp for headaches. Awapuhi is related to both white ginger and yellow ginger, but the latter varieties were introduced to the islands more recently.

The hiking grew increasingly difficult. "We have a choice," Zack told me at one point. "We can go up there"—he pointed to a thin trail of loose scree on the steep hillside beside us—"or we can stay down here on the floor of the valley and do the best we can." We determined that remaining on the valley floor would likely bring us into contact with more awa than the other route. Almost immediately after choosing the lower route, we ran into our first stand of awa. Four plants, each about 6 feet away from the others, stood in a shady spot in the woods, about 15 yards from the shallow river. "This is mahakea," Zachary told me. "I think most of the awa we will run into will be, because it's definitely one of the most common varieties in the forests." We took pictures, examined the health of the plants, cleared debris away from one, and moved on.

At one point I realized we were walking on feral *olena*, which is the Hawaiian name for turmeric (*Curcuma longa*), also a member of the ginger family. The brilliant orange rhizomes of olena were traditionally used to make fabric dyes, and the juice of the mashed rhizome was a staple remedy for earache and problems of the nasal passages. Zachary and I each pulled roots and broke them open to admire their colorful inner flesh. "There's so much out here," Zack mused. "I mean, I don't even know probably 1 percent of what's out here. But everywhere you turn, there are plants that are used for something. And lots of them are medicines."

As Zachary and I pushed our way through thick, thorny bush, we passed by different types of ti (*Cordyline fruticosa*). Probably originating from New Guinea, ti species were also introduced to Hawaii by Polynesians. The molasses-like cooked root is sweet, containing up to 60 percent fructose, or fruit sugar. In other parts of Polynesia, ti is made into a syrup in earthen ovens specially constructed for that purpose. In a 1789 journal entry published in the London book *A Voyage around the World*, author Captain Portlock reported encountering "tee" in Hawaii in abundance, and he apparently became so enamored with the plant that he brewed a beer from the cooked roots.

Traditional Hawaiians once valued the ti plant highly, using it for much more than the consumption of its sweet root. In battle, the ti stalk was used as a flag of truce. The leaves were braided and twisted to make sturdy sandals or tied in bundles for use as thatch on houses. Temporary ti leaf shelters made by hunters were called hale la'i. The leaves were commonly used as wrappers in cooking and also were laid upon food as matting to retain moisture in pit ovens called imu. At meals, condiments were typically placed on ti leaves.

Though ti leaves appear to possess little medicinal value, they were sometimes used as an expectorant in cases of cough or as a laxative. According to my close friend and expert in the native plants of the Pacific, Ariipaea Salmon, eating a quantity of the cooked root will quickly sober anyone who has consumed too much kava. "It will bring them right back, I mean right away," he commented. The leaves were the primary wrapping materials for poultices or hot stones employed in traditional treatments. Healers cooked packets of finely ground medicinal plants tightly wrapped in ti leaves over hot stones or immersed them in boiling water to magnify their healing properties.

Beyond its numerous secular uses, ti had occupied a prominent spot in the spiritual lives of traditional Hawaiians. Ti leaves served as charms against evil spirits and adorned the necks of priests as a sign of rank. Skirts of specially knotted ti leaves encircled the undulating hips of hula dancers, and were part of the decorative greenery laid upon the altar of the sacred halau hula temple, in honor of the goddess Laka. Menstruating women traveled with ti leaves wrapped around their ankles to mitigate the wrath of the volcano goddess Pele. In exorcisms, the possessed were laid upon ti leaves, and bunches of the leaves were slapped upon their bodies to dispel evil entities.

As we moved farther into the densely foliated throat of the valley, we came upon several muddy areas recently torn to pieces by wild pigs. The earth was gouged out in large patches, and surrounding bushes were completely trampled into the ground. Leading from these areas, pig runs wound into the forest, ending in thick bushes. The pig runs were easier going than beating through thick brush, and we walked along them when we could, looking and listening for any pigs that might be nearby. Several times we ran into brush so thick that we had to head back to the river's edge. Then we would either cross on logs suspended from bank to bank or jump across over rocks, hoping to find better hiking. In every instance, conditions were no better on the other side.

In one spot close to the water we came upon a magnificent patch of healthy taro. Broad, heart-shaped leaves rose 4 feet off the ground on thick, proud stems. Brought to Hawaii by Polynesians approximately 1,500 years ago, taro, also known as kalo, was important in Hawaiian diet and culture. Widely dispersed throughout the Pacific islands, taro (*Colocasia esculenta*) most likely originated in Asia, and it may have been cultivated in New Guinea 5,000 years ago or more. In the 1930s, botanist E.S. Craighill Handy recorded more than 300 varietal names for taro. The taro cultivars differ according to the color of the corm (the bulblike underground stem) or root, and the size, shape, and colors of the petioles (stems) and leaves.

The hard work of cultivation was central to the lives of the farmers who planted gardens of taro in both wet and dry areas. In the case of dry cultivation, forests were cleared and the broad-leafed taro was planted in beds, often in terraces laboriously hand-hewn into hillsides. In the wetlands of the numerous valleys of Hawaii, the plant was cultivated in mounds in man-made pondland patches known as lo'i. Traditionally, the Waimanu Valley was second only to the Waipio for wetland taro cultivation. Wetland taro grows more quickly than dryland taro, but both can remain in soil for up to 2 years after reaching maturity. This allows growers a great deal of flexibility with harvesting, and it enables people to use taro as they require it, not just when the plant needs to be pulled from the ground.

Hawaiians relied heavily on taro root as a staple, especially for making poi, which is similar to pudding. Poi was the starch food of choice among traditional Hawaiians, far more so than sweet potatoes or yams. To make poi, Hawaiians cooked taro roots fully, peeled them, and ground them on a concave board designed for that purpose. During the grinding, which was typically accomplished with a specially fashioned lava stone on a thick slab of hard ohia'a lehua wood, water was added bit by bit until the taro was smooth and sticky. Appearing at almost every meal, poi was eaten either fresh or a couple of days old and slightly fermented. Choosing one form over another was purely a matter of taste.

As a medicine, taro apparently enjoyed only limited use. Grated or scraped taro was employed in cases of pulmonary "consumption." It was also mixed with other plants and juiced to treat indigestion. Pieces of one variety of taro known as hoene were used as suppositories. But overall, the plant was much more a kitchen staple than an item of pharmacopoeia.

As Zachary and I made our way across slippery rocks, through almost impassable thorny bush, and along muddy pig runs deeper into the interior of Waimanu, we spotted several patches of tall, healthy taro. These were clearly not remnant gardens from planters long ago, nor patches of wild white taro, but current plantings in well-cared-for lo'i. "Yeah, you must have some guys who come in here and tend their taro," Zack commented as we encountered one large wetland taro patch with broad green leaves glistening in the sun. "These plants are in great condition." This was welcome evidence that some Hawaiians still cultivate taro. But for the most part, taro's days as a revered dietary staple are gone.

As the midday sun cooked the already steamy interior of Waimanu, Zachary and I came upon several patches of awa. In one very shady area, a dozen tall, healthy awa plants stood like sentinels. A couple of plants closer to the hill sprouted unusually thick stalks at least 12 feet tall. We took our time inspecting the various plants, and I shot several photographs. Zachary pointed through the bushes. "You see this hill here?" he asked. "What I think happened was that there is probably an old awa stand up on that hill. But over time, part of that hill slid down, and these awa plants sprouted up here. Probably those two big ones there were first, because you can tell they're old. Then stalks from those sprouted. I'll bet that none of these awa plants were put here by traditional villagers. Even the two oldest ones can't be more than 25 years old."

Fourteen or 15 different varieties of awa grow in Hawaii. Among the most popular and common of these are mahakea, nene, papa 'ele'ele, mo'i, and spotted hiwa. Each type of awa differs in the color of its stalks, leaf shape and color, and plant size. And because of differing ratios of kavalactones, the plant's

The author and feral awa in Hawaii's Waimanu Valley

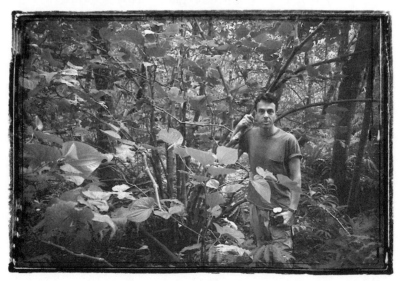

relaxing compounds, each differs also in the psychosomatic effects it imparts.

For the last 2 hours of hiking into the valley, we either followed the river along its bank or walked on stones in shallow water. It was slow, tough going. Zack and I were cut all over from tiny thorns, but the excitement of finding so many feral awa patches fueled our determination to press on. At one point, we peered into a clearing and spotted three very large, proud awa plants with glossy black stalks. We rushed to look closer. "You know, these are some of the nicest plants I've ever seen in the wild," Zack remarked. "Look at them. They're perfectly healthy. No leaf rot, no insects eating holes in the leaves and stems. As a farmer, you want your plants to grow this healthy."

We struggled up a long, slow incline and a bend in the river. Large mossy stones protruded from shallow, swift-moving water. An emerald river bottom of algae-covered rocks glistened under the bright midday sun. Just as we were about to stop to rest before turning back, we looked across the water and simultaneously beheld the single most magnificent awa plant we'd encountered all day. From atop a pile of large rocks at the river's edge, it presided in the manner of a throned monarch. A few stalks bent elegantly down toward the water, in a regal fan of dark green leaves. Several more interior stalks rose sceptrelike 12 feet in the air, displaying heart-shaped leaves burnished by sunlight filtered through a canopy of high trees.

Hawaiians speak of mana, or spiritual force. Mana is a primordial life power imbued in all living things, but especially concentrated in some. It is enhanced by rituals, practices, and natural forces. Ali'i, the chiefs, were considered to possess a great deal of mana. This was also the case with the kahunas, or priests. The halau hula, the temple of the hula, was possessed of great mana. Volcanoes definitely have very big mana. The Hawaiians also believe that mana can be conveyed in certain objects. A lei, for example, can carry the mana of the person who gave it. In the wild, certain trees or plants, by virtue of a majestic or imposing presence, are said to possess good mana. This awa bush at the river's edge had mana to spare.

Zachary and I shrugged off our packs, removed our sweat-soaked T-shirts, and rid ourselves of our sandals. We sat down, tired but elated, on large, mossy rocks in the water to take in the magnificent spot in which we found ourselves. Five hours into the valley, this recondite place at the bend of the river, with its fern-filled banks, mossy stones, and the grand awa plant, was the end of the trail that day.

We relaxed for about an hour, talking about Hawaiian awa and our extraordinary good fortune. All in all, we'd seen about 75 awa plants, most of them healthy and in good condition. "I've never gone this far into the valley," Zack mused. "But this is fantastic. Just think of how many awa plants we've seen out here, and how many more there must be even farther in by the mountains and on both hillsides." We agreed that in time, we'd return to explore other areas of the valley.

After resting up, we shouldered our packs and hiked back toward the ocean. Most of the way, we walked along rocks in the river shallows. The trek was slow, slippery, and hot, but in several places we found more wild fruit or discovered a few new patches of awa plants. Fruit juice, sweat, grime, and blood spots from thorn cuts stained our clothes, but we couldn't have cared less. At dusk when we stumbled into camp where suntanned

Hanna and Margaret were lounging contentedly, we looked like wild men from the deep forest.

KAVA, GROWN IN THE U.S.A.

Surf crashes loudly against the cliffs of the Hamakua coast, on the northeastern side of the Big Island of Hawaii. There the sea is rough. Wind blows almost constantly. The sun is hot and withering. The Pu'u'ala farm, whose name means fragrant hill, lies perched above the cliffs facing the rugged Pacific, and there the Gibsons wrestle with the forces of nature to grow awa. "We definitely could be trying to grow crops in an easier place, but we're here, and we're doing it," Zachary said. Pu'u'ala's land includes 595 acres owned by the Gibsons, plus another 150 acres leased from the Bernice B. Bishop Estate, the largest landholder in the Hawaiian Islands. When I was there, 55 acres were under cultivation. There were also 3 acres of nursery, an office, and a shed. The Gibsons have leased buffer zones of land on either side of the farm to prevent conventional farmers from moving in and contaminating the soil, water, and air with agricultural chemicals. "We don't want any chemical drift," Bill Gibson commented pointedly as we toured the grounds.

Before the sugar era with its swish of machetes through fibrous, syrupy stalks, the land where the owners of Pu'u'ala grow crops was a forest of proud ohia'a lehua trees. Traditional Hawaiians found versatile uses for the dark, hard, durable wood of the tree. Ohia'a lehua proved the ideal wood for fashioning canoes, building houses, and carving wooden bowls, boards, and temple artifacts. Thick, heavy slabs of ohia'a lehua were brilliantly transformed by artists into imposing sacred totems called ki'i, which stood 1½ to 5 meters tall. In honor of the goddess Laka, a branch of sacred ohia'a lehua was laid upon the altar in the halau hula. Vibrant crimson lehua flowers, favored by Pele the volcano goddess, were strung together on leis.

Kahala Ann Gibson is the inspiration behind Pu'u'ala. The land where Pu'u'ala farm stands today was owned by Kahala Ann's grandparents, who leased it to Hamakua Sugar for 100 years. "That was typical in those days," she told me. "The sugar companies had all the money, and the people had a lot of land but no money, so the sugar companies worked out all these sweetheart deals on land leases." When Hamakua Sugar went belly-up in 1994, Kahala Ann, an attorney, became determined to reclaim the land rights, and she suggested that the family start to grow native crops. The Gibsons won back their land rights, and Pu'u'ala was started.

Yang to Kahala Ann's yin, Bill Gibson provides the farm's financial and business backbone. Bill made his money in the high stakes fields of electronics and telecommunications. "An undertaking like this, the way we want to do it, requires a significant capital investment," he noted. Day-to-day operations and management of Pu'u'ala fall to Zachary, who supervises every aspect of work on the farm, from planting cuttings in the nursery to harvesting, cleaning, drying, and shipping.

Today, Pu'u'ala farm is home to 20 acres of awa, 16 acres of the Polynesian medicinal fruit noni (*Morinda citrifolia*), and 19 acres of neem (*Azadirachta indica*), an Indian tree whose various parts are used as antibacterial and antifungal topical agents. The farm is certified organic by HOFA, the Hawaiian Organic Farmer's Association. Making the decision to operate according to the sustainable practices and rigorous strictures required for organic certification was an easy choice for the Gibsons, who

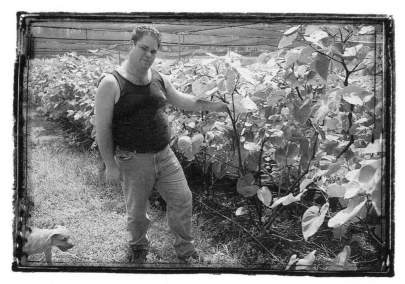

Organic awa grower Zachary Gibson and healthy awa plants

didn't want to pollute the land or adversely affect the people who worked there. "We really didn't have to think about it," Bill shrugged. "Once you understand the difference between farming with agricultural chemicals and organic farming, there's only one intelligent choice, and that's to farm organically. It's a harder path to take, but it's the only one that makes any sense at all. We want the land to remain healthy for generations."

The farm would not be able to operate if not for water from the Hamakua Ditch, which is 30 miles long and up to 10 feet wide. Every day an estimated 40 million gallons of pure water run through the ditch, which was constructed in 1910 to irrigate sugar fields. Water from the Hamakua Ditch originates in the Kohala mountains and runs right across the southwestern side of Pu'u'ala farm. This water is used for the farm's extensive irrigation system.

"I have two types of awa under cultivation here, mahakea and honakanaiki," Zachary told me as we perambulated a large awa field with rows of high, healthy plants. Mahakea, a fast grower with stalks that range in color from green to purple-black, is one of the varieties that has survived well in forests. Mahakea produces a large root within a couple of years, and the drink you get from it is a little bit peppery. The honakanaiki, with distinctive green stalks and raised dark spots, is considered one of the best drinking varieties of all types of Hawaiian awa. It's strong, with a smooth flavor.

The cultivation of awa requires cuttings of stalks from live, healthy awa plants. For Pu'u'ala's first cuttings, Zack trekked through the woods along the Hamakua coast, looking for feral plants. "When you find awa in a place that you can get to fairly easily, you prepare to take cuttings by tipping the plants back," he said. "It's pruning, but we call it tipping—cutting off the tops of the stalks. This results in new shoots that emerge from the stalks, and then you go back and take those, so you have really good, healthy stock for cultivation. But with awa plants that are really far away, like deep in one of the valleys, you can't keep going all the way there to prune and take a couple of new stalks. Instead, you take a couple of healthy stalks from each single plant, but not more. You can damage the plants by taking too many cuttings. You have to take just a few, and not be greedy." And, he said, you never, ever take any of the root. "Some guys go in and just destroy the plants, either by taking all the stalks, or just ripping the plants right out of the ground and hauling them away," he told me. "That's definitely not respect for the plants, or for the awa tradition. There are some guys running around calling themselves awa wild-crafters, and selling awa roots they've pulled. But that's not wild-crafting. They're just ripping plants out, and ripping off Hawaiians by destroying cultural treasures."

Some of the awa at Pu'u'ala grew from cuttings obtained in the Waipio Valley. Zack discovered a number of healthy awa patches there, and he brought bundles of cuttings back to the ranch for germination in the nursery. Additional awa was brought over from Hana, on the island of Maui. The Gibsons first planted awa in the nursery in 1995, and they planted their first field of 2 acres in December of that year. Pu'u'ala is now cultivating mahakea primarily because the variety has done well in the windy, sunny conditions of the farm.

The Hamakua coast, where Pu'u'ala grows awa at 200 feet above sea level, is windy and exposed. "Wind can really hurt awa," Zachary noted. "It will dry out your plants and make them vulnerable to insect infestation. So not only is irrigation very important, but you have to have windbreaks of tall trees grown thickly together. On the other hand, some wind is good because it agitates the plants and keeps a lot of insects away." The conditions at Pu'u'ala make growing awa appreciably more difficult. Awa was traditionally grown in a much more protected zone at an elevation of 2,500 feet, back away from the windy coast. "Those people had it easier for sure," Zack said.

Standing at one corner of the nursery where awa cuttings sprouted new plants, Zack explained that in the winter he and his crew make thousands of cuttings, and propagate thousands of plants. "Right now, we have about 40,000 awa plants in the ground," he said. "And that whole big field we were just in, that's 3-year-old awa, with big roots, just ready for harvesting." Zachary and his crew use organic fertilizers to build up the nutrition of the soil. They mix cinders and various soils for cultivation. Fast-growing trees provide shade to protect young awa plants from the hot sun. "When the awa plants are used to the sun, the shade trees are cut down and mulched and used to fertilize the rows," Zachary said. It's a self-regenerating system, with several strategies for building soil fertility and crop health. Irrigation, shade, weed mat, and lots of labor are required to keep the awa plants healthy. Weed cutting, mowing, and fertilizing are all accomplished by hand.

When Pu'u'ala was new, the Gibsons thought they would sell awa in bulk. They still do, but in 1998 they decided to produce a finished, boxed kava tea from leaf and stem cuttings. The leaves and stems in kava contain two active constituents, dihydromethysticin and dihydrokavain. In tea form, a small amount of these natural tranquilizers produces a peaceful feeling. The tea-making process begins with a harvest of about 50 plants at a time. The whole crew spends the entire day cutting the plants, cleaning them thoroughly with a power washer, and rinsing off any tiny dirt particles. "We go through all the leaves and stems very carefully," Zack said. "You have to get rid of all the tough, fibrous stalks, because they're lousy for tea." Once the good stalks and healthy leaves are separated out, they're cut up and packed on stands of perforated trays in a big walk-in dryer. "After about 4 to 5 days, they're completely dry and just perfect," Zack explained. "We pack the tea in dry containers, so it doesn't gather dust or moisture or develop any kind of bacterial problem. When you're processing a fresh, live product like organic awa, you have to think through every step."

With bulk awa and the kava tea to ship, Pu'u'ala stays busy. "These days, our dryer is humming all the time, usually 24 hours a day," Zack said. "You should see our electric bill. But the root comes out beautiful. Right now we have a couple of tons of beautiful, cut and dried 3-year-old organic awa root ready to ship, and at least 5,000 pounds of stems and leaves for tea."

After delivering his crash course on awa cultivation and processing, Zachary confided the personal rewards of his calling. "Being a Hawaiian awa grower is the most wonderful experience that could possibly happen to me," he told me. "I go out and roam around the hills and into the valleys, and I hunt awa. Basically, that's what I do out there. Then I come back to the farm and work on transforming that traditional awa into this certified organic dream. Cooking was my first real love in terms of work. But this is more than that. This is where I belong. Every Hawaiian wants to be really great at something. For some guys it's fishing or hunting. For me, it's growing awa."

In 1985, Ed Johnston hiked in the Waipio Valley and was captivated by the awa plants he saw there. He became a pioneer of modern Hawaiian awa cultivation, forming a special relationship with the plant that has become the central focus of his plant propagation career. "All I know for certain is that there's something very mystical about awa," he said. "Awa needs people to spread. I feel like I'm working for the plant."

Shortly after his valley experience, Ed received some awa cuttings from a friend and started growing the plant. He began to learn more about it, getting some of his knowledge from renowned awa expert Vincent Lebot. By early 1992, Ed Johnston's Alia Point Awa Nursery was the primary source for commercial awa cuttings in the Hawaiian Islands. "My first really big customer was Liloa Willard at Ho' Owaiwai Farms," he said. "He bought a lot of cuttings from me to get his operation going. Then Joel McLeary at Pu'u O Hoku Ranch on Molokai ordered cuttings from me and hired me to consult on propagation. Then C. Brewer, the big sugar company, hired me to advise them. Things have been going great guns ever since."

As Ed was telling his story, he, Zack, and I were rolling along a coastal road with two other experts who were spearheading the effort to cultivate awa on the Big Island of Hawaii— Jerry Konanui, the president of the Association for Hawaiian Awa, and Jerry O'oka, a University of Hawaii plant pathologist. "You're going to be very surprised by this place," Jerry Kona. ui told me, referring to our destination, Ho' Owaiwai Farms. Even as we drove up to the first high-tech greenhouse, I had a sense of what Jerry meant.

If Pu'u'ala sets the standard for organic Hawaiian awa, Ho' Owaiwai is its brilliant conventional counterpart. Set on 85 acres of arable land, Ho' Owaiwai was established by Liloa Willard, descendant of a whaler who married a native Hawaiian. Liloa's great-grandfather, James Campbell, helped to establish the Pioneer Sugar Mill in Lahaina, Maui. "Agriculture definitely runs in my family," he told us as we toured the greenhouse. Named after a mythical king of the Waipio Valley, Liloa got into awa cultivation in 1996. "We accepted an agricultural grant with matching funds and began to experiment with awa cultivation," he said. "The whole idea was to figure out how to create opportunity for small family farmers who were displaced by the collapse of the sugar industry here."

Liloa's son-in-law Tom Richmond, the farm manager at Ho' Owaiwai, proudly showed us the nursery where awa

Kava: What the Science Shows

Kava—the plant and the beverage—has been extensively studied, and its chemistry is well-documented. The medicinally active constituents are a group of resinous compounds known as kavalactones, or kavapyrones. While as many as 15 kavalactones are known, only 6 are found in kava to any significant extent: demethoxy-yangonin, dihydrokavain, yangonin, kavain, dihydromethysticin, and methysticin.

These kavalactones have been the objects of chemical research since the mid-1800s, and much is known about their mode of activity. They are muscle relaxants, and they act upon the limbic system of the brain to produce a pleasant feeling of ease and tranquillity. Hence, kava is a beneficial aid in the treatment of stress and anxiety.

A number of studies have demonstrated this. Here's a small sampling.

- In a double-blind, placebo-controlled study of 85 patients suffering from anxiety, those who were given a daily dose of 400 milligrams of one of the kavalactones—purified kavain—showed improvement in vigilance, memory, and reaction time.
- In a 4-week study of 58 patients experiencing anxiety, half were given 100 milligrams of 70 percent kavalactone extract three times daily, the rest a placebo. It was the kava extract group that experienced significant reduction in anxiety after just 1 week.
- In another study, 20 women with menopausal symptoms were given a daily 100-milligram dose of kava extract standardized to 70 percent kavalactone value, and 20 others with the same symptoms were given daily placebos. The control group experienced no change in symptoms, but the kava group had a significant reduction in menopausal symptoms as well as in anxiety and depression.

Out of many such studies have emerged some dosage guidelines for the use of kava as a safe alternative to prescription drugs for anxiety and insomnia. The most significant anti-anxiety studies show that an effective dose of kava contains between 70 and 210 milligrams of kavalactones. To promote sleep, a dose of approximately 200 milligrams of kavalactones 30 to 60 minutes prior to retiring is recommended.

cultivation begins at the farm—with tissue-culturing. Also called micropropagation, microcloning, and a number of other names, tissue-culturing is a painstaking process by which live tissue is removed from a plant and dissected under a microscope down to a tiny clean bud. When the process is repeated many times with tissue from the same plant, every plant that sprouts from these mass-produced buds will have identical growing characteristics and will, in turn, be used to yield even more sterile buds. "This gives us a huge number of identical plants, with exactly the traits we want," Tom told us as he hovered admiringly over trays in which thousands of perfect tissue-cultured awa cuttings sprouted in sterile white rock. "By controlling everything, we get exactly the varieties of awa we want, with just the right growing characteristics. And we get the cuttings ready for planting exactly when we want them." Zachary examined the expanse of the fine nursery greenhouse with its polished aluminum spans and flawless green netting. "Oh, man, I'd like to have this greenhouse," he enthused. Jerry Konanui shook his head with a laugh. "We'd all like to have this greenhouse."

Ho' Owaiwai Farms is employing the same kind of propagation research with other commercially viable crops, such as aloe, bromeliads, orchids, and antherium, so small family farmers can grow them as cash crops more easily. But Liloa's farm itself is no small family operation. Instead, rows stretching for several acres display healthy awa plants more than 10 feet high. The rows are manicured, and the plants rise out of perfect weed mat. Fungicides and pesticides are applied judiciously, at critical growth stages or when pests threaten the awa. Of course, pesticide use is not something I like—ever. Still, I recognize that many growers find it necessary. The owners of Ho' Owaiwai believe that their conservative approach to pesticide use is more economically viable and less labor-intensive than organic cultivation. "We're definitely trying to do this crop right," Tom said as the rest of us gazed down a long lane of flawless awa plants, witnessing firsthand the future of the Hawaiian awa industry.

In fact, traditional plots of a few healthy awa plants will not be the future of Hawaiian awa. The small stands of plants Zachary and I discovered in the Waimanu Valley are precious cultural relics of a Hawaii now long gone. They have little to do with what is in store for the awa industry. Nor will backyard family growers be the big recipients of income in the awa boom. Instead, the commercial victors will be the large growers, like Pu'u'ala, battling wind, sun, and heat, and Ho' Owaiwai, with acres of high-tech, tissue-cultured plantings. Former sugar giant C. Brewer is in the early stages of cultivating as much as a thousand acres of awa. All parties concerned firmly believe that awa will be a huge botanical product, and that strong market demand will drive an agricultural boom for Hawaii.

In the Hawaiian awa fields of tomorrow, tractors will roll along acres of neatly spaced rows, mechanically stumping plants one after another. Cleaning and preparing the roots will be an assembly line job, with pressure washers, sterilizing baths, and huge industrial dryers. And like the sugar plantations before them, the Hawaiian awa fields will crank out thousands of tons of the lucrative agricultural product of the day, this time for an eager world that is stressed out, anxious, and wired tight with information overload and work fatigue. That world needs the tranquillity that only this ancient, native plant can impart.

LAND
ETERNAL

You haven't been back to Baie Martellie in quite a while, have you?" Edouard Melsul pointed out the window of the Twin Otter aircraft as he spoke. Below, the splendid emerald hills of Pentecost Island rose up to meet us as we approached Lonorore, a grass airstrip on the coast. I nodded. "I'll be happy to see everybody again." Our conversation conjured in my mind the small village at the southernmost end of long, narrow Pentecost Island in the Republic of Vanuatu, where on my first visit in 1995 I had been greeted by the entire village, been shown tremendous hospitality, and made a number of friends. Edouard turned to me and said, "I think especially Michel will be happy to see you." Michel Bulliman, a big man in Baie Martellie, had looked after me during my previous stay, making sure I wanted for nothing. I was keen to see Michel again.

Named in 1768 by the seafaring explorer Louis Antoine de Bouganville, Pentecost Island features mountains that slope sharply down the long eastern and western coasts, leaving little habitable shoreline. Thus most of the people who live on Pentecost reside in the hilly interior. Edouard and I intended to travel down the western coast of Pentecost to the coastal village of Baie Martellie, which occupies one of the few big beaches on the island. We would stay with old friends, drink kava, and enjoy the spectacular scenic vista. There you can gaze past great rocky cliffs across a bay to Ambrym Island and its gigantic Maroum volcano, whose active, fiery cone illuminates the night sky with vibrant and brooding colors. From Baie Martellie, we planned to travel around the southern end of the island to the eastern coast, to villages where we would purchase kava. I brought a small day pack containing an extra pair of pants, a shirt, a camera, and film. Edouard carried a day pack containing a T-shirt, a sarong, a hanging scale, and a large pile of cash.

The Republic of Vanuatu, independent only since 1980, still walks on shaky legs. The tiny South Pacific archipelago of more than 80 islands, first visited by humans between 4,000 and 5,000 years ago, eventually became a joint colony of France and Britain dubbed the New Hebrides. When New Hebrides finally shook off colonial rule in 1980, the fledgling government inherited what a 1986 report called "a structurally imbalanced and impoverished economy." Vanuatu had a typical "plantation economy," with an expatriate-dominated, export-oriented agricultural sector existing simultaneously with poor subsistence farmers. The primary task of Vanuatu's new government was, in the report's words, to "articulate a comprehensive national development strategy to achieve productive economic transformation."

A former member of the Vanuatu parliament, and now a kava buyer, Edouard Melsul has devoted his life to the betterment of the Ni Vanuatu, the native islanders. In his parliamentary capacity, Edouard worked tirelessly to help improve life on the islands for the population of 175,000. Liked and respected by virtually everybody, Edouard the peacemaker helped to bridge opposing factions, which inevitably arose in the young, tiny coconut republic. Now, in his new role as kava buyer, he was communicating an upbeat idealism. "I think that this kava business can do very good things for all these people here," he told me. "They can live better, they can get the things they need, they can move forward. Kava is part of our tradition, so this will make people proud." I studied Edouard's bearded, dark chocolate face and his kind, wistful smile and felt fortunate to be in his company.

I, too, was arriving on Pentecost in a new capacity, as Vanuatu's Honorary Consul to the United States. In that post, I was focusing primarily on the kava trade. By stimulating demand for kava in the United States, I hoped to drive kava exports for Vanuatu, thereby doing my part for the country's economy. Other crops such as cocoa, coffee, and coconut made only modest money for a majority of growers. But kava offered the chance for small growers all over the islands to make an appreciably better wage.

In the United States, I had been working closely with Pure-World Botanicals, a large extraction company in New Jersey, on an ambitious program to develop superior kava extracts. I had conducted field research on kava in Vanuatu, from the planting to harvesting, drying, inspection, and export of the root, and helped PureWorld to identify trading partners. Scientists at Pure-World were able to turn the dried roots of Vanuatu kava into potent powdered and liquid extracts used by a number of major supplement companies.

Returning from my first travels to Vanuatu with an exciting story and more than 1,000 photographs, I worked with newspapers, magazines, radio, and TV shows in the United States to promote the benefits of kava and to stimulate demand for kava products. I wrote *Kava: Medicine Hunting in Paradise*, a book that chronicled the legend, history, and use of kava and its health benefits. In slide shows around the United States and eventually back in Vanuatu itself, I took viewers on a tour of kava culture. As a natural remedy for stress and anxiety, kava was good news. And the exotic, faraway place from which it came made kava intriguing.

The media ball began to roll with small articles and interviews in the fall of 1996. Ariipaea Salmon, the Tahitian prince who first took me to Baie Martellie, came to the United States to tour with me, promoting kava at trade shows and in the media. Many other people, from physicians to herbalists, were also vigorously promoting kava as the premier natural antistress, anti-anxiety remedy. As a result of this cumulative promotional effort, kava finally hit it big in February, 1998, with a feature article in the *Wall Street Journal*. A flurry of positive articles and interviews followed, and a kava segment on ABC's *20/20* was scheduled to air while I was back in Vanuatu.

Demand for kava products shot up like a rocket. Overnight, Vanuatu, with more kava in the ground than any place on Earth, was like the Wild West in the gold rush days. The islands were besieged by clueless foreign buyers who'd never set foot in a jungle before, tramping willy-nilly to small, remote villages, cash on their backs, to purchase kava. The market went insane. Edouard was philosophical. "Yes, it has been a very busy time," he said. "And too many people are trying to buy kava and causing confusion. But I still think the kava business will be very good for Vanuatu as time goes on."

But as things stood, Vanuatu, with its undeveloped infrastructure, was simply unable to meet the newly high demand. Now I was in Vanuatu again to help address that very issue—that is, to help improve the overall flow of kava out of the islands. By observing closely how kava was purchased from the growers, how it was then amassed into tonnage quantities, and how it was eventually moved to port and shipped to customers abroad, I could make some recommendations to agricultural agents in Vanuatu and to the country's chamber of commerce. There was a good chance that some logistical problems would be relatively simple and inexpensive to address. For example, on my previous trip to Vanuatu, I learned that members of one particular village could dry five times as much kava root if they had just a few rolls of wire mesh to use as racks, which I arranged for them to receive. But to see such solutions, I have to witness firsthand the entire chain of trade.

THE NAKAMALS OF BAIE MARTELLIE

After touching down, we spilled out of the cramped cabin with 18 other passengers, chickens, taro roots, and pineapples. We spotted our friends from Baie Martellie waiting for us—Michel and some others I knew from before. "How was your trip from the United States?" Michel asked. "Long, Michel. Long." The whole group clapped and hooted, as if it were the funniest thing ever uttered. Michel repeated "long" and shook his head, laughing. To them, America might as well have been another planet.

Just a couple hundred yards away at the shore, the boat of my nightmares waited for us. In that same red fiberglass shell with the 25-horsepower engine, no seats, and no life preservers, I had endured the scariest boat ride of my life during my first trip to Vanuatu. But as Edouard and I climbed in, the water looked relatively calm. With our small bags stowed under a plastic tarp in the foredeck and a friend named Jake at the outboard, we cruised slowly down the coast in clear turquoise water. Michel and another friend, Kami, smoked, and we all looked for sea life. A giant turtle and a large tuna swam nearby and quickly disappeared. Leno, another friend, pointed at the turtle with great excitement as it dove from sight. "Very good eating," Edouard commented. Atop high cliffs, giant bats known as flying foxes whirled in lazy circles around fruit trees. A gentle breeze blew, and the hot sun baked down on us.

We passed the small coastal villages of Hotwata, Panas, and Wali and pulled up to the beach by a cluster of coconut palms at tiny Panngi to drop off a bundle of taro for a family there. We continued down the coast as the breeze picked up—along with the chop. Salt spray blew at us in sheets, and we all shouted out in exuberance each time we were hit. The water got rougher as we approached Devil's Point. Named for its violent, swirling tides and large waves that crash furiously against high, rocky cliffs, Devil's Point extends like a finger at the southernmost tip of Pentecost Island. The tidal phenomenon at the point is caused by strong currents that stream down the western and eastern coasts of the long and narrow island, which measures 62 kilometers north to south and 18 kilometers east to west. At Devil's Point, the currents collide. On good days the point is rough, on bad days impassable. Though we were soaking wet by the time we rounded the point, we were in fact traveling on a very good day. As the seas calmed down and we wiped salt water from our faces, pristine Baie Martellie lay ahead, a wide crescent of unspoiled sandy beach, coconut palms, bamboo huts, green hills, a flowing freshwater river, and gentle, lapping waves. Paradise.

After landing on the beach and shaking hands with everybody in the village, Edouard and I were shown to our quarters, which were located in the back of a tiny makeshift store in a bamboo hut run by Chief Marcel. Behind tins of meat, boxes of tea, and bags of sugar and rice, we stowed our belongings on bamboo cots and made directly for one of the *nakamals* in the village.

Vanuatu's very name, which means land eternal, connotes the sense of ancient history and tradition of the islands. In the deeply rooted culture of the Ni Vanuatu, kava plays a central role in daily life. The nakamal is a hut set aside for kava preparation and drinking. In tiny Baie Martellie, three nakamals bustle with activity every afternoon and evening, as men gather to make and drink kava, talk, smoke, and enjoy each other's company. As we approached the nakamal, I heard the familiar toomp-toomp-toomp of freshly cleaned kava roots being pounded inside a wide pipe attached to a stump. Using a heavy pole, a man worked the standing pipe like a butter churn, smashing the kava with every heavy blow.

Freddie makes kava in Baie Martellie while Michel looks on

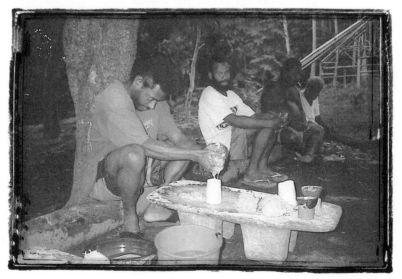

The late afternoon sun still shone, so for a while Michel, Kami, and Freddie, the village schoolteacher, made kava outside. The men piled freshly pounded root onto long, concave boards, hydrated the roots a little at a time, and kneaded the wet root mass by hand until it achieved the consistency of sloppy oatmeal. They scooped a handful of the mixture into a wide swath of palm fiber, then squeezed the mass until the juice ran out into a holding cup. When the liquid is strained through another piece of palm fiber into a coconut shell, the resulting fresh, potent liquid extract—superior to any other form of kava—is ready to drink. Its effects are usually immediately felt, and they last for hours.

In the village nakamals, people are called to drink one at a time, a process that goes on for hours. As a special guest, I was invited to drink first. Lifting a full coconut shell from Kami's board, I downed the kava at once and nodded my head in thanks. The others clapped. Even as I was putting the shell back down, the kava began to take effect. Michel informed me that we were drinking borogu, the most preferred variety of kava. Freddie the schoolteacher sat down beside me and asked how many shells I'd drunk: "Hameni shell yu dring?" he asked. As an answer, I pointed an accusing finger at Kami, and mimicked their pidgin: "Yu makem kava strong. Kilim hed." As the tropical sun set behind high cliffs, the "kava wave" washed over me. My limbs became relaxed, my muscles soft. My face became pliable as tension drained away. I felt thoroughly peaceful and at ease. A warm tropical breeze teased my face. Edouard sat shoulder-to-shoulder beside me, watching Kami. "I think they are making the kava especially strong tonight to welcome you back," he commented.

I drank kava with them for a couple of hours until I could take no more. Shortly after I bowed out of further rounds, a woman came to the entrance of the nakamal with a plate of fish, rice, and taro. Michel handed it to me. "What about everybody else?" I asked. Edouard smiled and patted my shoulder. "They know you can't drink too much, so you eat now," he said. "The rest of us will have a few more shells. Then we'll eat." The food tasted delicious, and I told them so. And, as happens with eating after drinking kava, the effects intensified. We sat chatting in Bislama, the pidgin national language of Vanuatu, as the night grew fully dark. Later on, when it appeared that my fellow kava drinkers had many more coconut shells ahead of them, I bid them "gud naet" and wandered off to the little bamboo store and lay down on a cot. I drifted off into blissful sleep, my last few fragments of thought ebbing away with the gentle lapping of waves.

The next morning, eight of us headed off barefoot into the bush toward a waterfall back in the hills. Walking along a freshwater stream flowing from the waterfall, we stopped to pick a papaya here, cut a stalk of sugar cane there. I carried a camera and a folding knife; the others carried machetes. Kami, noticing my knife, said, "When you leave, this knife stays, okay?" I agreed without hesitation. At a couple of deep spots in the stream, Kami and Leno slipped underwater and groped under submerged banks for freshwater prawns, which they loaded into a bag. "Fo lanch," Kami said with a broad smile.

In Vanuatu, the humidity stays around 75 to 80 percent, and the average daily temperature is between 70 and 80 degrees

Fahrenheit. The rainy season between November and April is very wet, and during the rest of the year rain showers are also common. The agreeable temperature and abundant moisture provide an ideal environment for plant growth. Still, the flora is limited in variety, especially compared with islands such as Papua New Guinea and the Solomons. Blame the relative geological youth of Vanuatu's islands, and the cyclones that rip through them during the rainy season. Another limiting factor is the soil composition. On Pentecost, weakly matured erosion-formed soil 2 to 3 meters deep supports all the flora on an island composed of 90 percent limestone.

Half an hour of brisk walking through lush forest of coconut, bamboo, guava, pandanus, hibiscus, and tree fern delivered us to the base of a high, roaring waterfall that crashed into a wide pool. In an instant, we were swimming and splashing. Then we hiked up a narrow, steep, and muddy path to the top of the falls and back into the interior of southern Pentecost Island, where miles of kava grow amidst papaya, cane, peppers, coconuts, bananas, and taro. We stopped here and there to examine kava plants and to take pictures, and then continued farther into the hills. As I gazed at miles of kava, I beheld the nation's treasury sprouting from the ground, embodying the hopes and dreams of the hard-working individuals who had planted every stalk.

Around noon we arrived at a small clearing. While a couple of the guys collected sticks for a fire, I went off with Edouard and Freddie to cut banana. By the time we returned, the prawns were all carefully wrapped in banana leaves and placed on the coals. The bananas and some taro brought by Leno were also quickly readied for the fire. As our lunch cooked, we ate juicy hunks of ripe papaya, chewed fresh cane, and talked about the kava trade. I explained that people in the United States were becoming aware of Vanuatu through the popularity of kava. That pleased my friends. We ate with our hands, sucking out the heads of the shrimp noisily, and throwing banana skins off into the bush. When the food was gone, we reclined on banana leaves and napped in the midday heat.

Early the next morning, Edouard, Michel, Jake, and I packed our gear under the foredeck of the red fiberglass boat. The ocean looked calm and the sky was clear. "I think we will have a very smooth passage to Baie Barrier," Edouard said, surveying the water. Home to a Catholic mission on the southeast coast of Pentecost Island, Baie Barrier would be our first kava-purchasing stop.

Reaching Baie Barrier required passage around three points—Guhunonbwe, Gousounanbouisil, and Batchil—all of which, like Devil's Point, featured churning tides and big surf. But the day was with us, and we arrived safely, if wet and salty. The sun shone hot and bright, with the glistening, densely foliated hills behind Baie Barrier reflecting light in a thousand greens. Several men sat on the beach with sacks of dried kava. "How did they know we were coming?" I asked Edouard. He made a circular waving motion south, in the direction of Baie Martellie. "Word goes from one village to the next," he said. "Many will come from villages all around this part of the island to sell their kava."

With the aid of a dozen villagers, we pushed the boat up onto the beach many yards past the high tide mark, roped it to a coconut palm, and unloaded our things. A couple of teenage boys wanted to carry my small pack, curious to see what it contained. I showed them a couple of knives, a flashlight, and my camera. That led to a photo session, with more teenage boys showing up, then younger children, and then a small crowd of young women. Pretty soon I was taking everybody's picture. Groups would huddle together, or jostle with each other, or make funny faces, or burst out laughing, or look serious—any of the things people do in front of cameras. Most of the villagers were happy and proud to be photographed. But several small children took one look at me and ran screaming for their mothers. Big scary white bogey man.

Edouard, Michel, and Jake set up shop in a nakamal on a rise overlooking the bay. Simple bamboo huts with palm thatch roofs perched on the hillside. Smoke from cooking fires rose through the roofs of several huts. People in the village, curious to see what was going on, peeked inside the nakamal to watch. Michel hung a scale from the center beam of the roof. Edouard sat on a plank, with a wooden box for a desk, and laid out a calculator, a pencil, paper, and a bag of cash.

Commerce with medicinal plants often goes like this. Small batches of herbal materials become larger batches, until there is enough of a plant to bring it to market or ship it for export. On the traditional islands of Vanuatu—where there are few or no roads, only occasional boats, and no significant infrastructure—the gathering of kava for export is inordinately labor-intensive. Small growers pick kava deep in the hills and carry the roots on their backs a few kilos at a time to their villages, where the roots are cleaned, cut, and dried in the hot sun. Over time, growers accumulate sacks of dried roots.

In this case, growers from the surrounding villages carried these sacks of kava on their backs, some for many miles, to sell to Edouard. That kava would later be taken back to Baie Martellie in the small red fiberglass boat and stored in a hut. Eventually, a couple of tons of dried root would be ferried off-shore, loaded onto an inter-island boat, and delivered to the Vanuatu capital of Port Vila. There the dried kava root would be pooled together a few tons at a time, inspected at the Tagabe plant quarantine station, and then air-freighted to extraction companies in the United States or Europe. When companies order 10 or 20 tons of dried Vanuatu kava root for extraction, they're usually completely unaware of the mammoth labor involved in meeting such orders.

By the time we were ready to begin weighing and purchasing kava, a small line of growers had formed at the entrance of the nakamal, each with one or two sacks of dried root. Each person gave his name, his village, and the varieties of kava in the bag. Michel opened each bag, reached deep inside, and pulled out a few large handfuls of root, checking to make sure no incompletely dried, soft, or molded kava was purchased. Michel, Jake, and I took turns hanging bags of dried kava on the hook of the scale, calling out the bag weights to Edouard, who calculated the number of kilograms times 800 vatu, the currency of Vanuatu. It came to a little more than $6 per kilo. Edouard dutifully noted all information in a log book, including the amounts paid. Every grower received cash on the spot plus a receipt. Several left with 50,000 or 60,000 vatu stuffed in the pockets of their shorts. The purchasing scheme generated a lot of kava, many satisfied growers, and a full set of fastidious records that would make the British proud.

Vanuatu's economy is based largely on the production and sale of agricultural products, including coffee, cocoa, and coconut. Almost all the commercially viable plants in the country were introduced, either by Polynesians or by expatriates. In the markets you can find bananas, citrus fruits and papaya, sweet potato, taro, chilies, and peanuts. Other fruits introduced to Vanuatu include avocado, carambola, guava, tamarind, mangosteen, litchi, pomegranate, fig, jackfruit, and mulberry. Vanuatu's growers are for the most part small shareholders who cultivate crops in limited quantities. Vanuatu is a tiny entity among world producers of those crops. Small, isolated, lacking infrastructure, and producing relatively low volume, the country and its growers can't hope to build wealth selling such commodities on the world market. But kava—indigenous to Vanuatu and part of its tradition for some 3,000 years—is a different story. The Ni Vanuatu are the world's most expert kava growers, filling hills and valleys and fields with strong, healthy kava plants. Virtually every young Ni Vanuatu begins to plant kava at around age 8, and continues to do so, often at a prolific rate, for life. Fiji sells more kava, but Vanuatu has considerably more in the ground. With few competitors at this point in time, Vanuatu can be a contender in the kava trade. It's the first crop in the nation's history that stands to make them some real money.

We slept that night on hard ground, covering ourselves with jackets to keep warm. In the morning after a bath in the river that runs down from the mountains into Baie Barrier, Edouard, Michel, Jake, and I consolidated the bags of kava into about 20 full, packed sacks. We loaded these in a great pile into the red fiberglass boat, tying them tightly inside a couple of blue plastic tarps. Sandwiching ourselves into the boat with the unwieldy cargo, we set off into the breezy morning. After a couple more days of kava buying farther up the coast, we headed back to Baie Martellie, our small boat groaning under too big a load of dried roots. From there, Edouard, Michel, and Jake boated me up to the Lonorore airstrip, where I wished them all farewell and caught a plane to Espiritu Santo, the largest of all the islands of Vanuatu.

PAEA'S NONI

When you're with Ariipaea Salmon, whom I know as Paea (pronounced "Pie-uh"), it's hard to be unobtrusive. For one thing, there's his hair—about 2 feet long, untamed, striated with gray, and impossibly thick. Then there's his barrel build, his bold traditional waist-to-ankle Tahitian tattoos, and his broad Mongolian-looking bearded face. His primary item of clothing is a colorful pareu, a wrap-around cloth. A pig-tusk bracelet is permanently fastened around his wrist. He stands out.

Of course, in Vanuatu, I don't exactly blend in seamlessly either. I'm white and a head taller than most Ni Vanuatu. Paea and I have several times appeared in Vanuatu's main newspaper, the *Trading Post*, sometimes on the front page. We've been the subjects of admiration and intrigue, and are known throughout the country. So we can't go anywhere on Santo or any other island in Vanuatu without a few people taking notice.

Under a trellis of hibiscus in a small patio café on the main street of dusty, collapsing old Luganville—the main town on sprawling Santo—Paea and I sat drinking cappuccino and talking about noni, or *Morinda citrifolia*. We might as well have been in a receiving line. Though we'd arrived only hours before, word got around that we were in town, and people we knew were dropping in nonstop. "Maybe we should go back to the hotel, so we can sit outside and talk," Paea suggested.

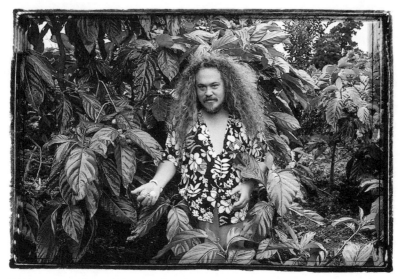

Tahitian prince Ariipaea Salmon and noni tree

Later, seated in the garden behind the buttressed concrete Hotel Santo, Paea began describing to me a grand vision for noni. "You know, Chris, ever since I was cured by noni, I have felt that at some point I would do something about this medicine, bring it to the world somehow," he said. "Now I am ready to do that." Paea spoke with a sense of great import, as though mountains were about to move and the sea would part for the passing of a momentous plan. "You see, noni has played an important role in my life," he went on. "Back in Tahiti, when I was a little boy, just 5 years old, I became very sick and would not recover, despite very good care. Eventually my condition became so bad that I was hospitalized in Taravao, in the southern part of Tahiti. My hands and legs and feet were all swollen, and there was blood in my urine."

Nobody could determine what was ailing young Paea, and that compounded the misery of his situation. The physician there, Dr. Turk, tried every conceivable treatment, but nothing worked. After a couple of months, his father took him out of the hospital and brought him home. "I didn't know it at the time, but my coffin had already been selected, and my grandmother had made a burial robe for me," Paea said. "You see, everybody thought I would die. But my father was very determined, and he took me to see two tahuas, the traditional healers who know all the plants and the ways to use them." The tahuas, an old man and woman, had Paea drink twice daily a very acidic-tasting beverage they made of crushed fresh noni fruits. From time to time they would add to it red ginger, also known as turmeric (*Curcuma longa*), metuapuaa (*Polypodium alternifolium*), and a few other herbs.

Paea, who had gone to these traditional healers almost at the point of death, began to improve. In a couple of weeks he was walking, and in a few months he was completely healthy and vigorous. "Dr. Turk believed that as a result of my ordeal, I would always have some kind of weakness in my system," he said. "He told my father that I would have many health problems later in life, and that I might be unable to father any children. My father would hear none of that. He was quite firm on the matter, telling Dr. Turk that I would grow up healthy and would father more children than any of my brothers. In all of this, my father was correct. I have the most children—11 of them—and six grandchildren. And I am still quite healthy at 46."

If I hadn't already heard the story a few times before, I would have stood up and cheered. But I already knew why Paea possessed a passion for noni. And who could blame him? Any plant that helps to heal so dramatically, albeit mysteriously, is sure to make a profound impression. Paea continued, "So you know, Chris, I have gone all over the Pacific islands learning about the healing plants, meeting the tahuas, living in Tahiti, Moorea, the Society Islands, the Cook Islands, Fiji, Tonga, Samoa, New Zealand, New Caledonia, and here in Vanuatu. I

What's Known about Noni

The Pacific islands' noni fruit is thought to be beneficial as an anti-inflammatory and anticancer agent as well as an all-around internal cleanser and general healer. Marketers have had a field day with noni, promoting its alleged usefulness in mitigating diabetes, cardiovascular disease, cancer, headaches, arthritis, and a host of degenerative diseases. All of this has stimulated market demand while making a mess of what's actually known about noni.

While the fruit and its preparations may turn out to be potently beneficial, the biochemistry of noni—or at least what is understood of it—goes only so far to justify some of these claims. The fruit certainly does contain a concentration of anthraquinones, which possess purgative activity. This may account for the "cleansing" effect described by many users. Certainly in cases of sluggish digestion and slow-moving bowels, noni can exert a stimulating effect, helping to increase peristalsis and cleanse the colon.

Noni fruit contains a concentration of vitamin A as well as the insecticidal octanoic acid. The presence of octanoic acid explains the traditional Hawaiian use of the fruit in insecticidal shampoos. Analysis shows the presence of numerous other acids, including linoleic, oleic, acetic, and palmitic acids.

The esters, ketones, lactones, and alcohols in noni are antimicrobial, anti-inflammatory, anti-carcinogenic, and immune-enhancing. Studies conducted on noni fruit demonstrate antimicrobial activity, including inhibition of both the *Candida albicans* virus and *Cryptococcus*, a cause of fungal pneumonia.

Noni appears to stimulate the production of T-cells, macrophages, and thymocytes, thereby enhancing immune function. And in animal studies, noni fruit extended the lives of mice with cancer. Subsequent analysis of the fruit shows the presence of a compound that possesses anti-tumor properties. Sedative, analgesic, and anti-inflammatory effects have also been noted.

Noni is a valuable medicinal plant, there's no doubt about it. Yet we have a great deal more to learn about what the plant contains and how it works. Considering the positive discoveries that have been made with noni fruit so far, there is excellent reason to think that further studies will prove the fruit and its preparations beneficial to health in numerous ways.

have walked all over these islands. You know about my interest in sandalwood, vanilla, and different products from the sea, and of course kava, which you and I have done so much work on together. But with noni it is more personal because in some ways, I owe my life to the plant. So for me, getting noni to people is a mission that I must fulfill."

I knew what was coming. Paea looked at me and said, "So the question is, do you want to be part of this?" In other words, did I want to get involved with noni, a traditional Polynesian medicinal plant, probably travel extensively throughout the Pacific islands with Paea, write and speak about the plant and its health benefits, and help to bring another beneficial botanical to a broader group of people, all the while having a great time? I laughed out loud and held up a hand for a high five. "I'm in." Paea broke into a big smile. "My psychic Helena said you would come," he said.

Paea had met some people who could back a noni venture, and he'd made a connection between a source for fresh, ripe noni in Tahiti and a freeze-drying facility in New Zealand. "I've been running all over the islands," he said. "And now I can tell you, I have found a way to make the very best noni product on the market." I didn't doubt it. If anybody I've ever met knows how to work with Pacific plants to make potent botanicals that deliver the desired effects, it's Paea.

Paea and I caught a beat-up Toyota Corolla taxi with all of its fenders bashed in, and we banged along pocked and rutted roads across dusty Luganville to see a Frenchman named Bernard Chardac. Operating out of a large metal shed on the outskirts of town, Bernard's business, Pacific Export, sells oil of tamanu, primarily to European companies. Tamanu's botanical name, *Calophyllum inophyllum*, means beautiful leaf, from the Greek *kalos* (beautiful) and *phyllon* (leaf). The tree is indigenous to Southeast Asia, but it's profuse in Polynesia, where it is traditionally known as ati. Tamanu grows up to 25 or even 30 meters in height, with long, spreading limbs. The tree trunk is typically thick with dark, cracked bark. The tamanu branches are covered with shiny, dark green oval leaves and small white flowers with yellow centers. The blossoms give off a delightful, sweet perfume. The fruit of the tree, about the size of an apricot, has a thin flesh and a large nut hull inside.

Tamanu wood is favored for making traditional handicrafts, bowls, boats, and houses. Considered sacred by Polynesians, the tree was also used for carving tiki, or idols of the gods. In Vanuatu, tamanu is known as *tamanu blong solwata*—tamanu of the sea. That's because it's dispersed by the seed-bearing fruits floating on the seas among the islands, washing up on shore, sprouting, taking root, and growing into trees. Hence, tamanu grows wild only in coastal areas, though it can be planted inland. The roots of the tamanu tree grow in coral sands beside the sea. And Paea insists that only those tamanu trees that grow in salty, coral sand have nuts that produce the highly prized medicinal oil.

Tamanu oil is one of the most remarkable plant derivatives in nature for its cicatrizing power—its capacity to promote the formation of new tissue, thereby encouraging wound healing. For this reason, it is a widely used traditional Polynesian topical medicine. Tamanu oil can be applied to cuts, scrapes, burns, insect bites and stings, abrasions, acne and acne scars, psoriasis, diabetic sores, anal fissures, sunburn, dry or scaly skin, blisters, eczema, and herpes sores. It can also be used to reduce foot and body odor. Tamanu oil is applied to the neck to relieve sore throat, and it's massaged into the skin to relieve neuralgia, rheumatism, and sciatica. Additionally, tamanu oil is a Polynesian beauty secret for promoting healthy, clear, blemish-free skin, and it's used by Tahitian women on their babies to prevent diaper rash and skin eruptions.

The oil of tamanu first came to the attention of researchers in the 1930s for its anti-neuralgic effects. Known in Fiji as dolno, tamanu oil was used to relieve the pain of sciatica, shingles, neuralgia, rheumatism, and leprous neuritis, for which it is remarkably effective. But its cicatrizing properties have received the most attention. In the medical literature on tamanu oil, several instances of its successful use in cases of severe skin conditions have been reported, with photographs showing before and after use. In one of the most remarkable instances, a woman was admitted to the St. Louis Hospital in Paris with a large gangrenous ulcer on her leg that would not heal. Though doctors were sure that amputation was inevitable, she was given regular dressings of tamanu oil. The wound eventually healed completely, leaving a smooth, flat scar. In other cases, tamanu oil has been employed successfully to heal horrible burns caused by boiling water, chemicals, and x-rays.

The oil of tamanu contains palmitic, oleic, and stearic acids, all three of which are common. The oil also contains a unique fatty acid called calophyllic acid, and a novel antibiotic lactone dubbed calophylloide. While the precise mode of tamanu's activity is yet to be established, calophyllic acid and calophylloide must play key phytochemical roles in the cicatrization and overall skin enhancement for which this remarkable oil is so effective.

The beneficial effects of tamanu oil—and its composition of unique constituents—aren't the only unusual attributes of

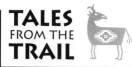

Coming Soon to a Natural Products Store Near You: Tamanu Oil

Tamanu oil, the natural all-purpose topical medicine from Hawaii, is not yet marketed in the United States and is for all intents and purposes unavailable on the mainland. But stay tuned, because I expect that situation to change shortly. I believe tamanu oil will be sold nationwide in the near future because of growing awareness of its broad healing powers. (See Resources on page 281 to learn how you can stay updated on the future of this oil.)

I personally use tamanu oil for a myriad of purposes, including cuts, sores, scrapes, bites, cracked and chapped skin, and abrasions. I will forever be in its debt for the great relief it provided me after a bad fall that injured my sciatic nerve, resulting in neuritis.

In my estimation, tamanu oil is a miracle agent, a botanical that lives up to each and every usage claim.

this Polynesian traditional remedy. Strangely, the nut kernel of the ripe fruit contains virtually no oil when it falls from the tree. Only after the nut kernel has been prized from its tough shell and carefully dried does it become rich in the luxurious healing oil. How this occurs is not understood. Approximately 100 kilograms of tamanu fruit yield a modest 5 kilograms of oil once this unusual alchemical process has taken place.

Bernard greeted us and gave us a brief tour of his shed. A small group of women sat on sackcloth on the cement floor. They broke the dark tamanu nut shells with hammers, throwing the shells into a pile and the nut kernels into a basin. Across the shed, tamanu nut kernels lay on drying racks. Paea pointed to some blond kernels. "You see here, Chris, these kernels are just freshly opened up," he said. "If you feel them or smell them, there's no oil. But now compare them with these over here." He pointed to trays of golden brown kernels sticky with oil. "If you pick these up and squeeze them, you get oil."

At a table, a Ni Vanuatu man was slowly pouring dark tamanu nut kernels into a small hand grinder. As he turned the handle, a golden green oil flowed from the grinder spout and into a containment vessel. "You see, it's all very natural," Bernard smiled. "There are no chemicals, no unnatural methods of any kind, and no heat. All we do is crack the nuts and lay them out. Nature makes them rich with oil by some completely mysterious process. Then we squeeze them through a simple grinder, a cold pressing, and we get the most beneficial healing oil. There is no need to add any chemicals. You simply bottle it, and you have nature's miracle medicine."

After a cup of coffee with Bernard and conversation about his hopes and dreams for the future of tamanu, Paea and I headed off back toward the main street in Luganville. "Did you like what you saw there?" Paea asked as we sauntered along. I told him that I did, and that I was keenly interested in the oil. "Good," he replied, nodding thoughtfully. "I knew you would like it. This oil is very important. I wanted you to see that, because when the time is right, I want us to be involved in tamanu oil too. Oh, man, there's a lot to do."

In early evening as the sun slid toward the horizon, Paea and I walked over to Lakirere, just around the corner from Hotel Santo. Lakirere was the brand-new nakamal of a friend of ours named Aaron Hegerfeld, from Hawaii. Unlike many nakamals, which are poorly constructed, unclean, or just shabby overall, Lakirere had an inviting atmosphere, tasteful construction, reassuring cleanliness, and a pretty garden atmosphere. Amidst the 90 other nakamals in Luganville, the place stood to do very well, and it was likely to pull in lots of expats and tourist divers. "You know," Aaron told us while reclining on a cushion in a breezy screened porch, "every night, my guys prepare kava from at least 70 kilos of green root, so there's a lot of kava being drunk here."

We walked outside to a shed where five young men were preparing kava from more than 70 kilograms of freshly harvested, cleaned, and ground kava root. Two sat before large rubber tubs filled with kava root and water, up to their elbows in the mixture. "These guys here are from Maewo," Aaron explained, referring to another island in Vanuatu. "See how thick the kava is? Nambawan, strong, strong. You like."

As if on cue, the night's crowd started drifting in, many on foot, some in cars. A number of Ni Vanuatu local government officials sat chatting on benches. Several Australians and Kiwis showed up, and eventually a contingent from the French agricultural research group CIRAD pulled in. Most notable among them was Vincent Lebot, the undisputed reigning guru of kava science and cultivation, accompanied by his wife Patrice and a Belgian nurse named Alicia. As night darkened and the stars brightened, the kava flowed, people lingered by the fire in the backyard, and the conversation included various schemes to improve conditions for the Ni Vanuatu and catch a piece of the kava business as it continued to grow. We drank coconut shells of kava for hours. Paea put an arm around my shoulder. "Are you glad to be back, Chris?" We both laughed aloud. I was glad to be back.

BOULEBAN'S GARDEN PARADISE

Denis Savoie, with his slender jeans, pencil mustache, and cowboy boots, could be a pistolero in a Mexican movie. Instead, he is the president of the Chamber of Commerce on Santo Island and grows taro commercially. Early in the morning, Denis sat in a rattling and dented Toyota truck outside the Hotel Santo. As Paea climbed into the passenger seat and I hopped in back, Denis gestured at his beat-up truck. "Still the same piece of crap World War II Toyota as last time," he laughed, yanking the truck into gear. Indeed, the last time I was on Santo Island, Denis had shown me around in the same truck, which stalled out several times and either had to be parked on a hill or left running.

We rumbled past the outskirts of town and set off for Fanafo, an area in the middle of the island, to visit a village whose people were eager to benefit from the kava business, and where one well-known grower was cultivating noni. As Vanuatu's largest island, Santo's 4,248 square kilometers make up more than 30 percent of the country's total land mass. Because of the island's size, its deepwater harbor, and its proximity to other strategically vital islands in the Pacific, more than half a million U.S. troops were stationed there during World War II, with an additional 10,000 Ni Vanuatu brought in from other islands to serve their needs. When the troops pulled out, they cleaned out hospitals, movie theaters, and office buildings, dumping a mountain of valuable remaining supplies—including trucks—into the sea. The Ni Vanuatu were left with roads that would become pocked and rutted, bridges that would rust and fall, broken tractors in the woods, and hundreds of corroding metal Quonset huts that would become overgrown mounds all over the island. Luganville, the bustling main port for a major

U.S. troop presence, would go to seed and become another forgotten, dilapidated, backwater tropical town off the beaten path.

We passed dense bush, patches of rain forest, stands of
giant banyan, great bamboo, and open grassland with scattered
shrubs. Morning glory and hibiscus broke up the rich green of
the landscape with purple and red. Coconut, coffee, and banana
grew here and there. Along an isolated stretch of dirt road, the
Toyota sputtered and rolled to a stop. Denis burst out laughing.
"Ol trak ia oli bagarap," he commented—this old truck is all bug-
gered up. After a couple of minutes under the hood with a
wrench and a cup of gasoline, Denis jammed the head of a
screwdriver into a hanging ignition and twisted, and the truck
shuddered back from the dead.

When we pulled into Fanafo, I was surprised to see that the
whole village had turned out to meet us. "I didn't tell you everything," Paea commented with a laugh. "There have to be some
surprises. These people are very happy to see you and me."
Everybody in the village stood together and sang a beautiful
greeting. Two women came forward and put spectacular floral
necklaces over our heads. We shook hands with a couple of village chiefs and then proceeded, with about 50 others, to a large
open nakamal. Men, women, and children crowded in. Seated
on narrow planks under a high palm-leaf roof, Paea and I waited
without speaking as one of the village elders stirred a bucket of
freshly made kava. Ten in the morning is early to start into kava,
but this was ceremonial, an offering of respect. The rest of the
villagers watched Paea and me. We were called up for coconut
shells of strong kava, which we drank right down. Then we returned to our planks and spent the next hour and a half up-
dating the villagers of Fanafo on the state of the kava business

around the world, and what increased demand in kava could mean to them.

Vanuatu's exports in kava have gone up tremendously in recent years. In 1995, Vanuatu exported 50 tons of kava; by 1998, that figure had climbed to 720 tons. Even so, many growers have yet to profit from the kava boom, and none in Fanafo had been solicited by any of the individuals and outfits that export kava. Still, they hoped that world interest in kava products would result in higher demand in Vanuatu, which in turn would mean that growers in Santo's interior would be able to sell more of their high-quality root.

Almost every area I visit has one grower who's known far and wide as being especially expert. In the interior of the island of Santo, a former schoolteacher named Bouleban is renowned for his impeccable plantings of healthy kava, ginger, chilies, and peanuts. Bouleban's farm, which he works with his wife and other helpers as needed, is considered a model for healthy crops. When I had met Bouleban on my last visit, he was supplying fresh kava roots to nakamals on Santo and in Port Vila, and generating a modest but steady stream of cash. Now he had begun a large orchard of noni. "You see, Chris, Bouleban has heard that noni will be very big," Denis Savoie said. "So he isn't waiting. When noni hits, he will be there with a good supply."

When we pulled up under a coconut tree beside a path leading to Bouleban's place, a mangy dog ran at us, teeth bared and snarling. We yelled back, and he skulked off head down into the bush. Moments later, Bouleban, followed by his wife and one son, appeared on the path. As we shook hands, he looked at me closely and said, "I know you. I can tell your name. Give me a moment." He thought for a few seconds and then continued. "Chris Kilham, correct? You were here 2 years ago."

Paea told Bouleban that we were eager to see how his crops were doing, especially the noni. "I have heard that noni will be a big crop someday as a medicine," he said. "The noni grows very well here, and we have plenty of land, so I have put in a couple hectares." That would be about 5 acres, which translates into a tremendous amount of labor—back-breaking clearing, soil preparation, and planting. Bouleban's agricultural ambitions seem matched only by his capacity to perform the work of several young men every day.

We walked over and around giant hills of ginger and rows of kava bushes, scallions, chile plants, and peanuts. Along the side of the field, under a makeshift tent to protect them from sun and rain, five women sat cleaning peanuts and placing them in a sack. Nearby dozens of healthy papaya trees stood heavy with fruit. "Wow, man," Paea said to Bouleban. "You did all this? This is unbelievable." Bouleban, unassuming in a stained T-shirt and grimy pants, gave the smile of a man who has accomplished something big and knows it. We cut ripe papaya from a tree and ate long, juicy slices. I snapped a small yellow chile pepper from a bush, popped it into my mouth, and bit down. I must have shown my surprise because Bouleban flashed a toothy smile and said, "Very hot peppers."

We rounded a dense corner of foliage to an orchard where noni trees, 18 months old and more than 2 meters high, hung with green and yellow grenade-shaped fruits. Bouleban, new to noni, was carrying on a tradition of cultivation dating back at least 1,000 years in the islands of the Pacific. Indigenous to Southeast Asia, noni (*Morinda citrifolia*) was domesticated and cultivated by Polynesians, first in Tahiti and the Marquesas, and eventually in the farthest outpost of their culture, Hawaii. Today, noni ranges from Tahiti to India and grows in the Caribbean, South America, and the West Indies. Its broad dispersal speaks of its value to traditional cultures.

The fruit of the noni tree has a distinctive and not altogether pleasant cheesy aroma. Nonetheless, noni fruit was traditionally eaten by native cultures in Samoa, Fiji, Burma, and Australia. In Hawaii and the Marquesas, noni was a famine food and was also fed to livestock. More commonly, the root and bark of the noni tree were employed as fabric dyes, a use for which noni remained popular in Polynesia, Asia, and Europe until the 1950s, when noni dyes were supplanted by cheaper synthetic dyes. Depending on the fixatives with which it was combined, noni was used to produce yellow, red, and purple colors. From Italy to India, noni dye colored carpets, sweaters, and turbans.

In traditional plant-based medicine, the fruit, flower, leaves, bark, and root of *Morinda citrifolia* have all been employed for diverse purposes. In Polynesia, noni leaves have a long history of topical use—either in poultices or mixed with oil—for the treatment of rheumatic pain, inflammation, neuralgia, ulcers, gout, cough and cold, boils, and ringworm. In Hawaii, the leaves were mashed together with other plants to heal wounds.

Actually, noni fruit was used relatively little in traditional medicine compared with other parts of the plant. But it was used. The Polynesians prepared the fruit for topical use, sometimes juiced and mixed with salt or sliced and applied to boils. In Hawaii, noni fruit was crushed and mixed with plants such as awapuhi and awa and applied to bruises, sprains, and swollen

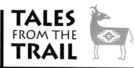

TALES
FROM THE
TRAIL

Which Noni to Choose?

In Polynesia, ripe noni fruit is put into a container, where it quickly decomposes and ferments. The pungent amber juice that remains at the top of the fermented fruit is consumed daily as a prophylactic, to enhance overall vitality and well-being. But most people cannot obtain fresh, fermented ripe noni juice. So what form of noni to use?

The active constituents in noni are volatile, which means that they are unstable and are easily reduced or destroyed by heat, light, air, moisture, and time. Currently, noni can be found dried and crushed, juiced and bottled, and freeze-dried. The processing method most likely to yield a beneficial noni fruit product is freeze-drying. The freeze-drying process is a stabilizing procedure that avoids destructive environmental factors, producing a stable material that retains a greater concentration of active, volatile constituents. (For information on finding a suitable noni product, see Resources on page 281.)

limbs. The Hawaiians also made a digestive by combining crushed noni fruit with cane juice. In addition, the fruit was part of cleansing formulas, which also included taro, cane juice, and other plants. By the 1930s, noni fruit was used more widely for internal purposes, including intestinal worms, fatigue, and respiratory disorders. Since that time, the juice of the ripe fruit has also been used as a folk remedy to help stabilize blood sugar in cases of adult diabetes.

After walking through Bouleban's fields, we sat on small wooden benches in the dark interior of his high-ceilinged bamboo hut and talked about kava and noni. "I have a steady market for kava right now, always to the same nakamals,"

Bouleban said. "And the markets take my papaya, green onions, chiles, and peanuts. Eventually, the noni will start to go. Right now is not yet the time. But when the time comes, I will have plenty of noni to sell."

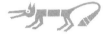

That evening all the regulars were back at the Lakirere nakamal. The young guys from Maewo had made the kava clean and strong, and Aaron was behind the bar moving shells of kava and making change as fast as he could. "So, Chris," Paea pondered, "tell me what you really think about this whole noni thing." I paused for a moment. "Well, it saved your life. That's a powerful thing. Lots of people use it, and they claim health results, and that matters a lot. And there's a great deal we don't yet know. But you're asking me if noni will be successful? Of course it will." Paea pulled at his beard and laughed. "I thought you would say that. Man, oh man, we have a lot of work to do."

We stood around outside with our friends and drank fresh Vanuatu kava for a couple of hours. At one point I wandered over to the fire by myself and gazed up at the sky. In the moonless night the stars gleamed brilliant and clear, radiant bursts of heavenly jewelry. I thought of my family and friends, and all the people I knew back home and would see again soon, and realized that far away on the other side of the world from them, in a remote archipelago, tiny dots on the great Pacific Ocean, I was viewing different constellations.

RESOURCES

The following information will assist you in finding the herbal products described in this book as well as help you to learn more about the field of botanical medicines. For great photographs of botanical expeditions and for recommendations on quality botanical products, see my Web site at www.medicinehunter.com.

More herbal products are available in natural food stores than anywhere else, but these products are increasingly found in pharmacies and supermarkets and on various e-commerce sites. Typically, natural food stores offer greater selection, more attentive service, and better-informed staff. While hundreds of companies manufacture herbal products, the following companies make herbal products that are generally easy to find in natural food stores. I am confident overall in the quality of products made by these companies and list them alphabetically. I have included their addresses and telephone numbers in case there isn't a good-quality natural food store that carries these products in your town. The omission of other companies is not a personal statement one way or another regarding the quality of their products.

Gaia Herbs
108 Island Ford Road
Brevard, NC 28712
Phone: (828) 884-4242

HerbPharm
P.O. Box 116
Williams, OR 97544
Phone: (541) 846-6262

Nature's Herbs
600 East Quality Drive
American Fork, UT 84003
Phone: (801) 763-0700

Nature's Way
10 Mountain Springs Parkway
Springville, UT 84663
Phone: (801) 489-1500

Planetary Formulas
23 Janis Way
Scotts Valley, CA 95066-3506
Phone: (408) 461-6317

Solaray
1400 Kearns Boulevard, Second Floor
Park City, UT 84060
Phone: (435) 655-6000

Yellow Emperor
P.O. Box 2631
Eugene, OR 97402
Phone: (541) 485-6664

Zand Herbal Formulas
1722 14th Street, Suite 230
Boulder, CO 80302
Phone: (303) 786-8558

The following categories of botanicals appear according to their order in the book.

AMAZONIAN BOTANICALS

Herbal products from the Amazon are relatively new to the market. A few companies do sell these items, however. Solaray offers catuaba, muirapuama, and guarana individually in capsules. They also have a sex-enhancing formula called ViraMax that combines these herbs with others. The Great Earth stores also offer these botanicals. The following three companies offer quality Amazonian botanicals as well, though their products are generally harder to find. In addition, Raintree has an excellent Web site with detailed information on Amazonian botanicals, at www.rain-tree.com.

Ashaninka Imports
P.O. Box 830662
Miami, FL 33283-0662
Web site address: www.ashaninka.com

Great Earth Stores
8981 Sunset Boulevard, Suite 103
West Hollywood, CA 90069
Phone: (800) 374-7328

NutraMedix
212 North U.S. Highway One, Suite 17
Tequesta, FL 33469
Phone: (561) 745-2917

AYURVEDIC BOTANICALS

Gaia Herbs, Nature's Herbs, Planetary Formulas, and Solaray all offer individual Ayurvedic botanicals as well as formulas. You'll find both curcumin and ashwagandha in these lines. The Ayurvedic category is just taking off. You will see many more brands and products over the next few years.

The Indus Valley Ayurvedic Center outside of Mysore, India, has a Web site. Check it out at www.Ayurindus.com.

MACA

Look for MacaPure standardized maca extract under the Great Earth, Sundown Herbals, and GNC labels. See my dosage recommendations in the maca section. Other good maca products include Solaray MacaMax shake, NutraMedix capsules and maca powder, and Bodyonics Adrenerlin. Click onto www.ViMaca.com as well.

KAVA

Much of the kava on the market today is worthless. Look for extracts of kava. Don't waste your money on ground-up kava root in a capsule. The minimum dosage of kava extract known to produce an effect is 70 milligrams of kavalactones. Many products fall far short of this. You will find extracts of kava in both powdered and liquid form. In my estimation, the following kava products are good quality and produce an effect: Great Earth

KavaQuil, Solaray Kava Kava Extract, Sundown Herbals Kava Kava Xtra, Source Naturals KavaPure soft gels, Gaia GBE Kava liquid extract, and HerbPharm kava capsules (these contain only 60 milligrams of kavalactones, so I would take two). Pu'u'ala farm makes a bagged kava tea, which produces a pleasant relaxing effect.

> **Pu'u'ala Farm**
> P.O. Box 391055
> Kailua-Kona, HI 96739
> Phone: (808) 329-8849

TAMANU

At the time of the completion of this book, nobody is marketing tamanu oil in stores. You can find the oil on Web sites, however. Stay tuned for further information on tamanu by checking my Web site, www.medicinehunter.com.

NONI

At present, the Great Earth stores alone offer a noni product using Paea's noni active freeze-dried material, which is the noni I use at home. As with tamanu, noni is relatively new to the market. You will see a plethora of noni products over the next couple of years.

BOOKS ON HERBS AND PLANT RESEARCH

Arvigo, Rosita. *Sastun: My Apprenticeship with a Maya Healer*. New York: Harper Collins, 1994.

Bruneton, Jean. *Pharmacognosy: Phytochemistry, Medicinal Plants*. New York: Lavoisier, 1995.

Davis, Wade. *One River*. New York: Simon and Schuster, 1996.

Duke, James A. *The Green Pharmacy*. Emmaus, Pa.: Rodale Press, 1997.

Evans, W.C. *Trease and Evans' Pharmacognosy*. 13th ed. Philadelphia: Bailliere Tindall, 1989.

Hoffman, David. *The Herbal Handbook*. Rochester, Vt.: Healing Arts Press, 1987.

Hoffman, David. *The Dictionary of Modern Herbalism*. Rochester, Vt.: Healing Arts Press, 1988.

Joyce, Christopher. *Earthly Goods: Medicine-Hunting in the Rainforest*. Boston, Mass.: Little, Brown and Company, 1994.

Kilham, Christopher. *Kava: Medicine-Hunting in Paradise*. Rochester, Vt.: Park Street Press, 1996.

Lamb, F. Bruce. *Wizard of the Upper Amazon*. Berkeley, Calif.: North Atlantic Books, 1974.

Leung, Albert Y., and Steven Foster. *Encyclopedia of Common Natural Ingredients Used in Food, Drugs, and Cosmetics*. New York: John Wiley and Sons, 1996.

Lewin, Louis. *Phantastica*. Rochester, Vt.: Park Street Press, 1988.

Murray, Michael. *The Healing Power of Herbs*. Ocklin, Calif.: Prima Publishing, 1995.

Plotkin, Mark J. *Tales of a Shaman's Apprentice*. New York: Penguin Books, 1993.

Samuelsson, Gunnar. *Drugs of Natural Origin*. Stockholm: Swedish Pharmaceutical Press, 1992.

Schultes, Richard E., and Robert F. Raffauf. *The Healing Forest*. Portland, Oregon: Dioscorides Press, 1990.

Tierra, M. *The Way of Herbs*. New York: Pocket Books, 1990.

Tyler, Varro, Lynn Brady, and James Robbers. *Pharmacognosy*. Philadelphia: Lea and Febiger, 1988.

Von Bibra, Baron Ernst. *Plant Intoxicants*. Rochester, Vt.: Healing Arts Press, 1995.

Werbach, Melvyn, and Michael Murray. *Botanical Influences on Illness*. Tarzana, Calif.: Third Line Press, 1994.

Wichtl, Max. *Herbal Drugs and Phytopharmaceuticals*. Boca Raton, Florida: Medpharms Scientific Publishers, 1989.

INDEX

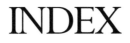

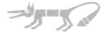

Underscored page numbers indicate boxed text. **Boldface** references indicate photographs.

A

Aarogyappacha (*Tricopus zeylanicus*), 167

Aattalaree (*Polygonum glabrum*), 153

Acai palm (*Euterpe oleracea*), 26, 31, 84

Adhatoda vasica, 120

Aloe vera, 122, 168

Amman pacharisi (*Euphorbia hirta*), 153

Andiroba (*Carapa guianensis*), 50

Annato. *See* Urucum (*Bixa orellana*)

Aripari (*Macrolobium acaciaefolium*), 50

Artemisia, 107

Ashwagandha (*Withania somnifera*), 122, **123**, 124–26, <u>125</u>, <u>151</u>, 167, 168, 284

Awa, 224–25, 226–27, 234–36, **235**, 237, 238, 240–45, **240**, 247–48. *See also* Kava

Awapuhi (*Zingiber zerumbet*), 230

B

Baie Martellie, Vanuatu, 226, 249, 250, 252, 253, 254, 255

Bangalore, India, 103, 110, 127, 132, 161

Black cohosh (*Cimicifuga racemosa*), 4

Boa Vista, Brazil, 55, 56, 57, 58, 59, 69, 73

Boswellia, 121

Brahmi (*Bacopa*), 168–69

Buriti (*Mauritia flexuosa*), 31, 98

C

Canawani, Brazil, 62, 69

Carapanauba (*Aspidosperma excelsium*), 25, 36, 77

Carhuamayo, Peru, 200, 204

Carimau, Brazil, 57

Cassava. *See* Manioc (*Manihot esculenta*)

Cassia ariculata, 152

Catuaba (*Erythroxylum catuaba*), 13–14, 22, 38, <u>52</u>, 53, <u>74</u>, 75, 76, 77, 78, <u>78</u>, 79, 83, 86, 92–93, 283

Caxiri, 65–69, **67**, 79

Cerro de Pasco, Peru, 189, 194, 196, 200, 201, 205

Chamomile (*Chamamelum nobile*), <u>35</u>

V

Vanuatu, 225–26, 249, 250, 251,
  252, 253, 255, 259, 260, 262,
  263, 265, 273, 275
Vassourinha (*Scoparia dulcis*), 44

W

Waimanu Valley, Hawaii, 220,
  226–27, 248

Waipio Valley, Hawaii, 220
Water hyacinth (*Eichornia crassipes*).
  See Muru
Woolly foxglove (*Digitalis
  lanata*), 5

Y

Yanahuanca, Peru, 201, 202